Handbook of Acupuncture
in the Treatment of
Musculoskeletal Conditions

Biographical details

Lü Shaojie is Chief Physician and Director of the Acupuncture Department, Xiangyang Hospital, Henan Province. He was born in 1956 to a family which had practised traditional Chinese medicine for generations. He studied under his father and the direct supervision of Dr. Cheng Xiangsheng, Professor of the Xiangfan Medical School, subsequently graduating from Hubei College of Traditional Chinese Medicine with a degree in Chinese Medicine. He then became a doctor in the Acupuncture Department of Xiangyang Hospital. Now with more than 20 years of clinical experience, Doctor Lü has undertaken much clinical research in TCM, especially in relation to treatment of the sequelae of cardiovascular diseases, spondylosis and pain. He has published a number of books including *Acupuncture in the Treatment of Nervous Diseases* and *Acupuncture in the Treatment of Orthopaedic Diseases*.

Li Zhaoguo is the Director of the TCM English Centre and Associate Professor at the Shanghai University of TCM. He graduated from Xi'an Foreign Languages University in 1982, subsequently studying for a master's degree under Shao Xundao, Professor of Medical English at Xi'an Medical University, and a PhD in Acupuncture at Shanghai University of TCM under the supervision of Professor Li Ding. Li Zhaoguo has published a number of books on the use of English for TCM as well as compiling two dictionaries and translating many books.

Robert J Dickie, FRCGP, DRCOG, BMedBiol graduated from Aberdeen University in 1978. After lecturing in pathology for some years, Dr. Dickie then underwent training to become a General Practitioner. Since 1985, he has been a full-time GP on the Isle of Lewis, with particular interests in dermatology and forensic medicine. For many years he has practised homeopathy and acupuncture and offers these services to patients in his NHS practice. He is also involved in training medical undergraduates and postgraduates both in the UK and overseas.

Handbook of Acupuncture
in the Treatment of
Musculoskeletal Conditions

Lü Shaojie

Chief Physician and Director, Acupuncture Department
Xiangyang Hospital, Henan

Translated by

Li Zhaoguo

Director, TCM English Centre
and Associate Professor of Shanghai University of TCM

Consultant medical editor

Robert J Dickie

FRCGP, DRCOG, BMedBiol

Donica Publishing Ltd

Note

Medical knowledge is constantly changing. As new information becomes available, changes in treatment, procedures, equipment and the use of drugs become necessary. The editors/authors/contributors and the publishers have, as far as it is possible, taken care to ensure that the information given in this text is accurate and up to date. However, readers are strongly advised to confirm that the information, especially with regard to drug usage, complies with the latest legislation and standards of practice.

Although every effort has been made to indicate appropriate precautions with regard to acupuncture treatment, neither the publishers nor the author can accept responsibility for any treatment advice or information offered, neither will they be liable for any loss or damage of any nature occasioned to or suffered by any person acting or refraining from acting as a result of reliance on the material contained in this publication.

Copyright © 2002 by Donica Publishing Ltd

First published 2002

ISBN 1 901149 00 5

British Library Cataloguing in Publication Data
A catalogue record for this book is available from the British Library

Commissioning editor Yanping Li
Managing editor Rodger Watts
Illustrator Maggie Pang

Typeset by Aarontype Ltd.
Printed in the UK by CPI.
The publisher's policy is to use paper manufactured from sustainable forests.

Contents

Chapter 3 Upper limb conditions

Chapter 4 Lower limb conditions

Editor's foreword

Acupuncture has made great strides in the West in the past 30 years and has now become established as a widely accepted therapy in a variety of contexts. Its use as an effective treatment in the management of pain is well documented. However, the difficulties faced by Western acupuncturists in studying original Chinese-language texts have restricted access to the wealth of experience gained over the centuries by doctors in China, the home of acupuncture.

It was therefore with a mixture of curiosity and excitement that I tackled the task of editing this book, which adopts an integrated Chinese-Western approach to the assessment and treatment of a range of musculoskeletal conditions. It was a fascinating and enriching experience to discover the similarities and differences in the description of the symptoms encountered and to understand how the disparities between Chinese and Western society, although narrowing rapidly, are reflected in the circumstances in which certain disorders occur. In these and other instances, notably in terms of examination techniques, it was necessary to adapt the text in places to harmonize the clinical features and to conform to standard Western clinical practice.

The long-established tradition of acupuncture in China means that patients there generally have more awareness of the type of treatment involved and are possibly more tolerant of the techniques utilized than many patients in the West. As a result, I deemed it necessary to add notes at certain points so that the acupuncturist can advise the patient what to expect in terms of needling sensation and the length and anticipated benefits of acupuncture therapy. Similarly I inserted reminders about important anatomical structures which may be encountered during acupuncture treatment in order to ensure that the procedures remain safe at all times. These various amendments to the original text have been made in consultation with the author.

As the editor of this book, it is my hope that it will be of benefit to fellow practitioners in helping them to treat a variety of musculoskeletal conditions, achieve a better understanding of the advantages of acupuncture for these conditions, and offer an effective and safe therapy to their patients. I am grateful to the author for allowing me the opportunity to be involved in this project.

Stornoway
September 2001

Author's foreword

Acupuncture is an indispensable part of traditional Chinese medicine and has a history of over four thousand years. It continues to be used extensively in clinical practice. Acupuncture treatment is especially applicable to the treatment of musculoskeletal and soft tissue conditions, where it is particularly effective. Many of these conditions cannot be satisfactorily treated by drugs due to the large number of side effects and the high cost of treatment. Acupuncture treatment is inexpensive, highly effective and has no side effects.

I began to practise acupuncture in 1971. After treating thousands of patients and also experimenting with techniques on my own body, I have been able to draw up a systematic analysis of the practical use of acupuncture in the treatment of musculoskeletal and soft tissue conditions, partly based on assessment by modern medical diagnostic methods.

In writing this book, I made a careful study of the writings of the great doctors throughout history and drew on the experience of my teachers. Combining this with a modern and realistic approach to the subject, I investigated each disorder and acupuncture point, consulting a variety of sources of clinical material and data. It is my sincere hope that this book will offer readers a new perspective on the treatment of musculoskeletal and soft tissue conditions, thus enabling them to improve the effectiveness of the treatment of patients.

This book could not have been written without the constant support and encouragement of Liu Yunzhen and Wei Jiarang, current and former presidents of Xiangyang Hospital, and my wife, Zhou Yucui. I am deeply indebted to them.

Xiangyang
April 2001

Introduction

This practical handbook presents the author's unique clinical experience in the assessment and acupuncture treatment of 63 musculoskeletal and soft tissue conditions and also provides valuable clinical notes offering an insight into the treatment involved.

This pioneering work, the first of its kind in the English language, is intended for doctors and other health professionals whose main training is in Western medicine, but who also apply acupuncture as a complement or supplement to Western treatment methods. It can also be used by doctors and health professionals who have an interest in discovering the benefits of acupuncture in the treatment of musculoskeletal conditions, but who do not practise such therapy themselves; in other words, they can consult this book to decide whether and when to refer a patient for acupuncture treatment for a musculoskeletal condition, can appreciate the likely results of such treatment, and can take this into account if and when further treatment using Western medical methods is required to improve the condition or complete a cure. In general, all acupuncturists will be able to benefit from study of the clinical symptoms and manifestations in order to use the treatment techniques and point selection discussed for each disorder.

In the West, the growing library of texts in English has provided instruction on acupuncture, diagnostics, pattern differentiation and treatment strategies, but a consistent corpus of specialist acupuncture texts in English has yet to be developed. The author therefore offers this book as a contribution towards building up such a group of works by illustrating how acupuncture functions in a specialist area.

The interest in acupuncture in the West has increased rapidly in the past 30 years. When Western doctors first heard of acupuncture it was greeted with a certain degree of scepticism. Over the succeeding decades, the scientific basis of acupuncture has become accepted and its applicability within the context of conventional Western medicine has been established. In the UK, many doctors now practise acupuncture both in primary care and (to a lesser extent) in secondary care settings. Its value in the management of pain has become widely accepted and it is presently offered as a powerful and effective therapy.

It is instructive to note that traditional medicine in China nowadays is tending towards the adoption of a pragmatic approach to the treatment of most types of diseases and disorders. This means that many of the more recent generations of doctors practise a type of medicine that can be considered as a synthesis of Western and Chinese medicine. In this context, it appears that a proportion of the traditional diagnostic methods that were part and parcel of traditional Chinese medicine (TCM) are being neglected in favour of a more Western approach to diagnosis. Many of the older generation of doctors in China do not support this trend, which has also met stiff opposition among TCM practitioners in the West.

Nevertheless, certain aspects of the present situation in the health sector in China tend to suggest that it is unlikely that this trend towards integrating Western and Chinese medicine will be reversed in the near future. In the first place, TCM and Western medicine are seen as two sides of the same coin in China. All doctors undergo the same basic training in medicine, subsequently specializing in TCM or Western medicine. Therefore, both types of medicine are considered as mainstream, with none of the overtones of "complementary" or "alternative" with which TCM is labelled in the West. As a result of their thorough and complete medical training, acupuncturists in China are schooled in the use of techniques that require expert guidance that is possibly harder to find in the West at the "grass-roots" level.

Secondly, nearly all doctors in China work in hospitals or in clinics within hospitals. This enables greater specialization even at the GP-equivalent level, but also results in a need to see large numbers of patients every day. It is this as much as anything that has caused a shift away from the more time-consuming TCM diagnosis to Western techniques. The greater availability of more expensive medical equipment has also favoured this movement.

However, even where these two factors have resulted in greater attention being paid to Western diagnostic techniques, many doctors and patients still prefer to rely on TCM for the provision of remedies. The clinic set-up and the accessibility of medical care mean that patients will frequently see their doctor on a daily basis until their condition is cured. In addition, the thorough grounding all doctors receive in medical theory and practice allows them to display much greater confidence in needling to a greater depth than is usually the case for Western practitioners of acupuncture. This higher frequency of visits and greater depth of needling is also accepted (and even expected) by patients in China. It does, however, make it more difficult to transfer treatment styles directly from China to the West.

As a result, this book includes certain modifications to the treatment that would be applied in China. These modifications relate principally to the depth of needling. Safety aspects and medicolegal considerations in the UK mean that great caution must be used when needling near to blood vessels, nerves, body cavities and joints. In situations where there are potential problems with the depths of needling used in TCM, the depth has been reduced to minimize danger whilst at the same time maintaining clinical efficacy. Practitioners wishing to perform the techniques described in this book must follow safe clinical practice at all times: this includes employing single-use disposable needles and minimizing the risk of introducing infection from the skin surface.

In this book, the frequency of treatment remains at the level at which it would be practised in China. Clearly, there are a variety of reasons impeding many patients in the West from attending the clinic every day. In such cases, treatment will take longer to have an effect than if acupuncture is carried out every day.

In a number of instances, acupuncture treatment needs to be supplemented by other therapies, notably corticosteroid injections and exercise. It should be noted in the UK context that injections of corticosteroids or other substances at acupuncture points can only be carried out by health professionals specifically authorized by their qualifications to do so. This would not normally include TCM acupuncturists, unless they have the necessary medical qualifications for administering injections.

Patients should always be encouraged to take a responsible attitude to their health and appropriate exercises are often an invaluable aid to completing a successful course of acupuncture treatment.

This book is divided into four chapters according to the part of the body involved. Each condition or disorder starts with a description of its symptoms and clinical manifestations. The descriptions of clinical conditions, including the causative factors for these conditions, may vary a little from those in Western medicine textbooks but will give practitioners an insight into the way in which TCM practitioners in China understand, assess and manage a range of clinical problems. In this context, the investigations suggested by the author have been edited to conform to currently accepted UK practice.

For each condition, the section describing the symptoms and clinical manifestations is followed by a table detailing the acupoints (acupuncture points) to be selected to treat the condition and the type of needles to be used. For each acupoint, the depth and direction of needle insertion are specified. Unless specifically stated otherwise in the text, needling directions are always given relative to the skin surface. Perpendicular needling therefore indicates insertion at an angle of 90° to the skin surface and horizontal needling indicates insertion parallel to the skin surface through the subcutaneous tissue after the dermal layer has been penetrated. Other angles of insertion are stated in the text.

Standard acupuncture points are designated by the letter and number coding used in the National Acupuncture Points Standard of the People's Republic of China issued by the State Bureau of Technical Supervision. The locations of non-standard points, in particular those related to tender areas, are described in greater detail. The appendix contains a number of diagrams illustrating the location of all the points used in the book. The practitioner must know how to locate the acupoints accurately and should always take account of the anatomical structures that may be encountered during acupuncture. It is the responsibility of the acupuncturist to ensure that needling will not impinge on or damage important structures such as nerves, joints, blood vessels and internal organs. When needles are inserted, the patient will experience a particular needling sensation at each acupoint; this is indicated for each point in each section. It is good practice to advise the patient of the type of sensation they are likely to experience.

Following the table relating to acupoints, there is a description of the method to be followed in administering acupuncture. This indicates the position to be adopted by the patient, the length of time the needles should be retained, the nature and extent of needle manipulation, whether electro-acupuncture is suitable, whether cupping therapy[1] is to be applied when the needles are withdrawn, and the length and frequency of treatment and the interval between repeated courses of treatment.

The clinical notes provide information on the effectiveness of acupuncture treatment for each condition, the optimal time for such treatment, the existence of any contraindications, and additional therapies to support acupuncture.

It is hoped that the treatment principles described in this book will go some way towards furthering understanding of the role that acupuncture can play in treating a variety of musculoskeletal conditions.

---

[1] Cupping therapy is performed by using heat to create a vacuum in specially designed small glass cupping jars, which are then inverted and attached by suction to the skin at the appropriate acupoint(s).

Chapter 1

Disorders of the head and neck

1 STIFF NECK

Stiff neck is a syndrome of neck stiffness and pain manifesting itself after sleep. There are two major causes. The first is an improper sleeping position, where the head is kept turned to the side for a lengthy period, or where the pillow is too high, too low or too hard; this leads to spasm of the cervical muscles. The second cause is the neck being exposed to a draught or lying on a cold object during sleep, giving rise to unilateral spasm of the cervical muscles after a certain time.

Clinical manifestations
- often occurs in young and middle-aged people
- usually sudden onset
- stiff, sharp pain when the head is moved to one side, backwards or forwards
- the patient turns the body to look to the side
- points of obvious pain are indicated at the origin or insertion of the sternocleidomastoid muscle or the trapezius and longus capitis muscles

TREATMENT
Acupoints and techniques

Combination of points	Needles used	Insertion technique	Needling sensation
Luozhen point (on the affected side): Located on the point between the second and the third metacarpal bones and 0.5 cun behind the metacarpophalangeal joint (see diagram, page 163)	No. 32 filiform needle, 1 cun in length	Insert slightly obliquely perpendicularly upwards (at an angle of 75°) to a depth of about 0.5 cun (care should be taken not to puncture too deeply)	Distending pain in the palm

Luojing point (on the affected side): Located on the neck, on the medial point of the line connecting Tianrong (SI-17) and Tianchuang (SI-16) and on the medial point of the upper part of the sternoclei-domastoid muscle (see diagram, page 165)	No. 30 filiform needle, 1.5 cun in length	Insert to a depth of 0.5-0.8 cun towards the spinal column	Distending pain in the neck

Method
- The patient adopts a sitting position.
- The needle is first inserted into Luozhen. When a heavy, distending sensation is felt, the needle is manipulated with large amplitude and at high frequency, and the patient is asked to move the neck slowly towards the affected side.
- Manipulation of the needle continues until neck movement is pain-free, then the Luojing point is needled with the needle being retained for 20 minutes.
- Before withdrawing the needle, another session of manipulation takes place.
- Acupuncture is performed once a day until the stiff neck is completely cured.

Clinical notes
This needling therapy is extremely effective in the treatment of stiff neck. If treatment is given on the day the stiff neck first occurs, the Luozhen point only is needled as described above with strong stimulation; the patient is asked to move the neck to the affected side until alleviation or disappearance of the pain. The needle is retained for 20 minutes, during which time it is manipulated once. In most cases, the patient is relieved of the pain or cured after just one session.

A small number of patients need two or three acupuncture sessions. The Luojing point is added for the second session. The Luozhen point is needled first as described above; the Luojing point is then needled with mild stimulation. The curative effect of this treatment for patients without cervical spondylopathy is relatively satisfactory.

2 SPASMODIC TORTICOLLIS

Spasmodic torticollis, or spasmodic wry neck, results from a powerful, involuntary contraction of the cervical muscles, which produces a twisting of the neck and an unnatural position of the head due to dystonic contraction of the sternocleidomastoid and trapezius muscles.

The aetiology of spasmodic torticollis is not clear. It is considered that the dominant precipitating factors are emotional, and some authorities believe that the disorder is caused by organic lesions in the corpus striatum or the thalamus.

Clinical manifestations
- often seen in adults, without marked sex predilection
- peak age of onset is about 40; more than two-thirds of patients are in the 30-50 age range
- also seen in children and the elderly
- onset is usually slow and progresses gradually, although abrupt onset can also occur
- at the early stage, the majority of patients feel a force pulling the head towards one side or unconsciously incline their head to one side
- in mild cases, the extent of muscular spasm is limited; the onset is unilateral without myalgia
- in moderate cases, onset is bilateral with mild myalgia
- in severe cases, nearby muscular groups (chest, back, shoulder and face) are involved in addition to bilateral muscles, and the disease has a tendency to spread with severe myalgia
- the dystonia increases with walking and standing, and is reduced by stimuli such as touching the neck or chin

TREATMENT
Acupoints and techniques

Combination of points	Needles used	Insertion technique	Needling sensation
Fengchi (GB-20, bilateral)	Two no. 30 filiform needles, 2 cun in length	Insert quickly and push towards the contralateral GB-20 for about 1.6 cun	Distending pain and/or pain radiating upwards

Fengfu (DU-16)	No. 30 filiform needle, 1.5 cun in length	Insert perpendicularly towards the great occipital foramen for 0.3-0.7 cun	Local distending pain
Dazhui (DU-14)	No. 30 filiform needle, 1.5 cun in length	Insert slightly obliquely perpendicularly upwards (at an angle of 75°) to a depth of 0.5-1.0 cun	Local distending pain
Neiguan (PC-6, bilateral)	Two no. 30 filiform needles, 1.5 cun in length	Insert towards Waiguan (SJ-5) to a depth of 0.5-1.0 cun	Regional distending pain and/or pain radiating to the dorsum of the hand and middle finger

Method
- The patient adopts a sitting position.
- The acupoints are needled with the needles being retained for 40 minutes; during this period, the needles are manipulated once after 20 minutes.
- After the needles are withdrawn, cupping therapy is performed at DU-14 for one minute.
- Acupuncture is performed once a day for ten consecutive days (one course of treatment).
- Recommence the treatment after an interval of five days, if necessary.

Clinical notes
Generally, the manifestations of spasmodic torticollis are not very significant at the early stages and are usually neglected. Once the disorder is discovered or diagnosed definitely, it has usually been present for some time. As a result, it will also take a long time for the treatment to be effective. It will normally take at least ten sessions before any tangible benefit is felt. The duration of treatment depends on the severity of the disease and the patient's sensitivity to acupuncture. Usually, severe cases (with symptoms at the back, chest, shoulder and face muscles) need longer treatment. In mild cases with involvement of the cervical muscles only, the treatment period is short and the effects relatively good. During and after treatment, the patient should be advised to undertake some physical exercise in order to consolidate the therapeutic effects.

3 INJURY TO THE ERECTOR SPINAE MUSCLE IN THE CERVICAL REGION

Injury to the erector spinae muscle is caused by prolonged immobility of the neck, such as when sitting in one position when writing, working in front of a computer or watching television, or when carrying a load on one shoulder or on the head. In cases with a history of obvious trauma, the factors mentioned above may exacerbate the disorder, especially when the weather changes suddenly, such as on cloudy, rainy or snowy days.

Clinical manifestations
- sudden onset when the head is turned after rest or is bent, for example to look for something
- pain usually involves the 6th and 7th cervical vertebral area; the pain is not severe at the beginning, but worsens within one day, especially when turning the head
- pain worsens, radiating to the back, shoulder and throat, when the head is turned slightly or the neck is bent
- no pain when the head and neck are maintained in a fixed position
- in severe cases, neck and head support is required when getting out of bed

TREATMENT
Acupoints and techniques

Combination of points	Needles used	Insertion technique	Needling sensation
First tender point: Located at a point 0.5 cun lateral to the midline of the 6th cervical vertebra	No. 30 filiform needle, 1.5 cun in length	Insert perpendicularly to a depth of 0.5-0.8 cun towards the transverse process	Local distending pain, radiating to the same side of the 3rd thoracic vertebra
Second tender point: Located at a point 0.5 cun lateral to the midline of the 7th cervical vertebra	No. 30 filiform needle, 1.5 cun in length	Insert perpendicularly to a depth of 0.5-0.8 cun towards the transverse process	Local distending pain, radiating to the same side of the 3rd thoracic vertebra

Luojing point (on the affected side): Located on the neck, on the medial point of the line connecting Tianrong (SI-17) and Tianchuang (SI-16) and on the medial point of the upper part of the sterno-cleidomastoid muscle (see diagram, page 165)	No. 30 filiform needle, 1.5 cun in length	Insert to a depth of 0.5-0.8 cun towards the spinal column	Distending pain in the neck
Hegu (LI-4, on the affected side)	No. 30 filiform needle, 2 cun in length	Insert to a depth of 1.0-1.5 cun towards Houxi (SI-3)	Regional distend-ing pain

Method
- The patient adopts a sitting position.
- The acupoints are needled with the needles being retained for 40 minutes; during this period, one session of gentle needle manipulation takes place.
- Acupuncture should be performed once a day; one course of treatment consists of six sessions.
- An interval of three days is required between two courses of treatment.

Clinical notes
Some of the symptoms of stiff neck and injury to the erector spinae muscle are similar. They can be differentiated as follows: stiff neck is worst at the onset and is often unilateral; although injury to the erector spinae muscle may occur at the same time as stiff neck, the pain gradually worsens and radiates out to the shoulder and back.

Effective results may be obtained with acupuncture in cases where there is mild osteophyte formation of the cervical vertebrae; in cases accompanied by severe osteophyte formation or intervertebral disc prolapse, patients are advised to consult Western medical specialists.

4 DISORDERS OF THE TEMPOROMANDIBULAR JOINT

Disorders of the temporomandibular joint may be caused by such factors as prolonged unilateral chewing, straining to bite hard objects, or trauma to the joint. The shallowness of the temporomandibular joint socket and any abnormal changes affecting it, prolonged weakness of the patient's constitution, insomnia, and rheumatoid arthritis tend to lead to the onset of such disorders.

Clinical manifestations
- commonly seen in young people
- pain and snapping noise on the affected side while chewing
- restricted opening of the mouth
- migraine may occur as a complication
- vertigo, tinnitus, numbness of the tongue, and dryness of the mouth
- in severe cases, difficulty in opening the mouth and chewing
- X-rays may show changes in the temporomandibular joint

TREATMENT
Acupoints and techniques

Combination of points	Needles used	Insertion technique	Needling sensation
Xiaguan (ST-7, on the affected side)	No. 30 filiform needle, 1 cun in length	Insert to a depth of 0.3-0.5 cun along the articular cleft	Distending pain around the temporomandibular joint
Taiyang (EX-HN-5, on the affected side)	No. 30 filiform needle, 1 cun in length	Insert obliquely downwards (at an angle of 45°) towards the jaw to a depth of 0.5 cun	Regional distending pain
Hegu (LI-4, on the affected side)	No. 30 filiform needle, 1.5 cun in length	Insert to a depth of 0.5-0.8 cun towards the wrist	Distending pain in the thenar eminence

Method
- The patient adopts a sitting position.
- The acupoints are needled with the needles being retained for 40 minutes; during this period, one session of needle manipulation takes place.
- Acupuncture should be performed once a day; one course of treatment consists of six sessions.
- An interval of three days is required between two courses of treatment.

Clinical notes
Acupuncture is quite effective in treating disorders of the temporomandibular joint at an early stage. In cases where a snapping noise occurs and the patient finds difficulty in opening the mouth, consideration should be given to combining local corticosteroid injection with acupuncture for an effective result. If both the above treatments fail, orthodontic splinting may be considered.

5 TENSION HEADACHE

Tension headache is a type of chronic headache caused by long-term muscular contraction and vasoconstriction at the head, face, neck and shoulder. The headache results from persistently contracted muscles.

Clinical manifestations
- generally begins after the age of 20 with women more commonly affected than men
- pain frequently starts from the neck or temporal region, manifesting as a feeling of compression, heaviness, distension or tension
- pain can persist for several days, weeks or even months
- frequent, often daily, attacks of non-throbbing, bilateral pain
- at the late stage, pain or tenderness may occur at the neck or shoulder or the exit of the greater occipital nerve at the occipital region
- tension of the skin and subcutaneous tissues at the neck
- in some patients, pain may be induced by extension and flexion of the head

TREATMENT
Acupoints and techniques

Combination of points	Needles used	Insertion technique	Needling sensation
Taiyang (EX-HN-5, bilateral)	Two no. 30 filiform needles, 1.5 cun in length	Insert obliquely (at an angle of 45°) towards GB-8 for 0.3-1.0 cun	Distending pain in the temporal region
Shuaigu (GB-8, bilateral)	Two no. 30 filiform needles, 1.5 cun in length	Insert horizontally towards the occiput for about 1.2 cun	Local distending pain
Fengchi (GB-20, bilateral)	Two no. 30 filiform needles, 2 cun in length	Insert towards the spinal column for about 1.6 cun	Local distending pain and/or pain radiating to the ipsilateral temporal and occipital regions

| Neiguan (PC-6, bilateral) | Two no. 30 filiform needles, 1.5 cun in length | Insert towards Waiguan (SJ-5) to a depth of 0.5-1.0 cun | Regional distending pain and/or pain radiating to the dorsum of the hand and middle finger |

Method
- The patient adopts a sitting position.
- The acupoints are needled with the needles being retained for 40 minutes; during this period, one session of needle manipulation takes place.
- Acupuncture is performed once a day for six consecutive days (one course of treatment).
- Recommence the treatment after an interval of three days, if necessary.

Clinical notes
Acupuncture has specific effects in the treatment of tension headaches. Pain can be eased or relieved in three to five sessions in most cases when the tension headaches are of recent onset. Where cases with a history stretching back several years have significant tender points or painful nodules at the neck or shoulder, these should also be treated by acupuncture. Although the course of treatment is comparatively long in such cases, relatively good therapeutic effects can also be obtained.

6 CLUSTER HEADACHE

Cluster headache is a common headache syndrome. Unlike migraine and tension headaches, cluster headaches are always unilateral, occurring at the orbit and temporal area.

Clinical manifestations
- seen more frequently in men than women
- usually begins between the ages of 20 and 50
- attacks may be precipitated by tobacco and/or alcohol
- usually occur on the same side for an individual patient
- commonly occur at night, awakening the patient from sleep, and recur daily in a cluster period of weeks or months
- headaches may begin as a burning sensation over the lateral aspect of the nose or as pressure behind the eye; ipsilateral photophobia, lacrimation, ptosis and nasal congestion are common
- attacks are severe, and last from 10 minutes to 2 hours

Examination
- significant tenderness at the superior part of the orbit
- pain may ease when the tender point is pressed

TREATMENT
Acupoints and techniques

Combination of points	Needles used	Insertion technique	Needling sensation
Yangbai (GB-14, on the affected side)	No. 32 filiform needle, 1.5 cun in length	Insert towards Yuyao (EX-HN-4, the midpoint of the eyebrow) for about 1.2 cun	Local distending pain
Toulinqi (GB-15, on the affected side)	No. 30 filiform needle, 2 cun in length	Insert superiorly and horizontally towards Muchuang (GB-16) for about 1.5 cun	Local distending pain

Taiyang (EX-HN-5, on the affected side)	No. 30 filiform needle, 2 cun in length	Insert towards Touwei (ST-8) for about 1.8 cun	Local distending pain
Yifeng (SJ-17, on the affected side)	No. 30 filiform needle, 1.5 cun in length	Insert towards the medial and posterior aspect of the mandible for about 0.5-1.0 cun	Local distending sensation and pain

Method
- The patient adopts a sitting position.
- The acupoints are needled with the needles being retained for 40 minutes; during this period, one session of needle manipulation takes place.
- Acupuncture is performed once a day for six consecutive days (one course of treatment).
- Repeat the treatment when the headache recurs.

Clinical notes
The therapeutic effects of acupuncture for treatment of cluster headache are reasonably good; pain can generally be relieved or eliminated after three sessions or so. Local corticosteroid injection can be tried for the few patients who do not respond to acupuncture therapy. After being cured, the patient should be advised not to smoke, drink alcohol or eat spicy or irritating food. If the headache recurs, repeat the treatment.

7 MIGRAINE

Migraine manifests as severe and repeated headache, generally unilateral. It is characterized by sudden onset of severe headache, which may resolve spontaneously or with drug treatment without sequelae, and recurrences after variable periods when the patient is free from headache.

In most cases, the condition is associated with psychological factors, endocrine disturbances, or dietary or environmental factors. The frequency of occurrence may vary from several times in one day to once every few months.

Clinical manifestations
- may occur at any age and can start from childhood
- morbidity increases with age and reaches a peak at 30-50 years, before gradually declining
- in most cases, the condition occurs initially in patients under 30, 50% of whom have a family history of migraine
- clinically, it is characterized by sudden onset, remission and recurrence

Prodromal stage

The prodromal stage is variable and may include the following features:
- about half an hour before onset, a scintillating scotoma or fortification spectrum may occur on the side contralateral to the headache and gradually increases in size; sometimes this is accompanied by ipsilateral hemianopia
- there may be general malaise, disturbance of speech, numbness of fingers and lips, dizziness, pale complexion, or polyuria

Headache
- after the prodromal symptoms disappear, a throbbing headache occurs suddenly, often located on one side of the frontal or parietal region
- the headache may spread across the head, increasing gradually in severity
- the headache is often accompanied by retrobulbar pain, photophobia, phonophobia, teichopsia, nausea or vomiting
- the climax can last for two to three hours and the pain then gradually subsides

Post-headache stage
- after the headache resolves, the patient often feels tired or may experience excitement, euphoria or an empty feeling in the head

TREATMENT
Acupoints and techniques

Combination of points	Needles used	Insertion technique	Needling sensation
Taiyang (EX-HN-5, on the affected side)	No. 30 filiform needle, 1.5 cun in length	Insert obliquely (at an angle of 45°) towards GB-8 for 0.3-1.0 cun	Distending pain in the temporal region
Shuaigu (GB-8, on the affected side)	No. 30 filiform needle, 1.5 cun in length	Insert horizontally towards the occiput for about 1.2 cun	Local distending pain
Baihui (DU-20)	No. 30 filiform needle, 1 cun in length	Insert obliquely (at an angle of 45°) towards the bone for about 0.5 cun with the tip of the needle pointing slightly backwards	Local distending pain
Fengchi (GB-20, on the affected side)	No. 30 filiform needle, 2 cun in length	Insert towards the spinal column for about 1.6 cun	Local distending pain and/or pain radiating to the ipsilateral temporal and occipital regions

Method
- The patient adopts a sitting position.
- The acupoints are needled with the needles being retained for 40 minutes; during this period, the needles are manipulated once after 20 minutes.
- Acupuncture is performed once a day for six consecutive days (one course of treatment).
- Recommence the treatment after an interval of three days, if necessary.
- Repeat the treatment when migraine recurs.

Clinical notes
Acupuncture is a specific treatment for migraine and the pain can be eased or relieved in most cases within around 10 minutes after insertion of the needles.

Patients generally do not want to complete the course of treatment, but should be advised to do so in order to prolong the period of remission and decrease the severity of recurrence. If the patient comes to the acupuncture clinic for treatment immediately the attack occurs, the condition can be cured (with no further recurrences) after several sessions. If acupuncture fails after six sessions, or if the condition worsens, it is necessary to consider whether the diagnosis is correct. In this situation, the cause of the headache should be ascertained by re-evaluating the history and examination and treated accordingly.

Chapter 2

Disorders of the trunk

8 INTERCOSTAL NEURALGIA

The main symptom of intercostal neuralgia is pain in a band-shaped area along the distribution of the intercostal nerves caused by stimulation of one or more of these nerves.

Clinical manifestations
- history of trauma, sprain or contusion
- existence of a primary disease, such as rib fracture, tumour, osteophytosis of the thoracic vertebrae, spondylitis, tuberculosis, pleural lesion, furuncle, boil, sore or ulcer at the nerve root
- in mild cases, pain radiates along one or more intercostal spaces during coughing or violent sneezing
- in severe cases, radiating pain occurs when the patient breathes deeply, coughs, sneezes or yawns, or when turning over in bed; the pain may interfere with sleep

Examination
- a fixed or variable tender point can be found at the relevant intercostal area in the majority of cases
- in cases with injury, a marked oedematous area with tenderness can be found at the initial stage
- X-ray may show degenerative changes in the thoracic vertebrae, spondylitis, fracture of the rib or pleural lesion

TREATMENT
Acupoints and techniques

Combination of points	Needles used	Insertion technique	Needling sensation
Neiguan (PC-6, on the affected side)	No. 30 filiform needle, 1.5 cun in length	Insert towards Waiguan (SJ-5) to a depth of 0.5-1.0 cun	Regional distending pain and/or pain radiating to the dorsum of the hand and middle finger

Yanglingquan (GB-34, on the affected side)	No. 30 filiform needle, 2 cun in length	Insert towards the space between the tibia and fibula for about 1.8 cun	Local distending pain
Tenderness: Two tender areas are located on the sensitive site in the intercostal region	Two no. 30 filiform needles, 2 cun in length	Insert in the selected tender points and push horizontally and anteriorly along the intercostal space for about 1.8 cun	Local distending pain

Note: When needling the tender area, the proximity of the pleura to the skin surface, particularly in thin individuals, must be remembered.

Method
- The patient adopts a sitting position.
- PC-6 and GB-34 are punctured first.
- Ask the patient to inspire deeply or cough while strong stimulation is applied to both needle shafts simultaneously after insertion.
- This procedure should result in the pain being eased. The tender areas are then punctured with the same needle manipulation stimulation applied as for the initial points.
- The needles are retained for 40 minutes.
- Cupping therapy is applied for one minute at the chest immediately after the needles are removed.
- Acupuncture is performed once a day for six consecutive days (one course of treatment).
- Suspend the treatment if the intercostal neuralgia is cured in less than six sessions.

Clinical notes
Acupuncture has a remarkable effect in the treatment of intercostal neuralgia. Satisfactory therapeutic effects can be obtained very quickly in most mild cases or cases with unilateral intercostal neuralgia in the space between the 4th and 5th ribs. Relatively satisfactory therapeutic results can also be obtained in secondary intercostal neuralgia if the primary lesion has been eradicated. In long-term obstinate cases, the above method should be combined with drugs; good therapeutic effects can also generally be achieved in such instances.

9 OCCIPITAL NEURALGIA

Occipital neuralgia is a general designation referring to neuralgia of the greater occipital, lesser occipital and great auricular nerves.

The main causes of the condition are the common cold, otitis media, local infection, occipital trauma, spondylitis of the 1st-4th cervical vertebrae or sleeping on a pillow that is too hard.

Clinical manifestations
- the disease is often seen in young males
- commonly occurs after the common cold or trauma
- at the initial stage, pain is limited to the region innervated by the greater occipital nerve (the occipital and posterior parietal region)
- one or two days later, the pain is aggravated, sometimes with severe attacks
- in most cases, pain is spontaneous or precipitated by movement of the head or coughing and sneezing
- in severe cases, pain may also occur at the regions innervated by the lesser occipital and great auricular nerves
- the pain is aggravated when lying down and eased when sitting up

Examination
- an obvious tender point can be found below the occipital tuberosity about 2 cm lateral to the median line at the involved side
- in severe cases, a markedly tender point can also be found at the mastoid process region

TREATMENT
Acupoints and techniques

Combination of points	Needles used	Insertion technique	Needling sensation
Fengfu (DU-16)	No. 30 filiform needle, 1.5 cun in length	Insert perpendicularly towards the great occipital foramen for 0.3-0.7 cun	Local distending pain

Naokong (GB-19, on the affected side)	No. 30 filiform needle, 1.5 cun in length	Insert towards Fengchi (GB-20) for about 1.3 cun	Local distending pain
Tender area (on the affected side): No fixed location but selected by eliciting tenderness or pain around Fengchi (GB-20) below the occiput on the affected side	Two no. 30 filiform needles, 1.5 cun in length	Insert and push towards the spinal column for about 1.3 cun, one needle along the border of the occipital bone and the other along the posterior aspect of the sterno-cleidomastoid muscle below the occipital bone	Local distending pain

Method
- The patient adopts a sitting position.
- The acupoints are needled with the needles being retained for 40 minutes; during this period, one session of needle manipulation takes place.
- Acupuncture is performed once a day for six consecutive days (one course of treatment).
- Suspend the treatment as soon as the condition is cured.

Clinical notes
Occipital neuralgia is a common condition, and is often misdiagnosed as cervical spondylosis or posterior headache induced by fatigue. A relatively satisfactory effect can be obtained if an accurate diagnosis is made. The patient should be advised to use a soft pillow, not to work for prolonged periods and to deal with stresses and other psychological factors in order to avoid a recurrence of the disorder. For obstinate cases with long-term neuralgia and no therapeutic effects after six sessions of acupuncture, local corticosteroid injection can be used; this technique can achieve relatively good therapeutic effects.

10 DISORDER OF THE THORACIC VERTEBRAL JOINTS

Disorder of the thoracic vertebral joints is a back and chest pain syndrome caused by such injuries as extensive bending of the thorax when loading heavy objects, children falling out of bed, one shoulder touching the ground with torsion of the thorax, or striking the side of the thorax and back in sporting activities.

Clinical manifestations
- mild unilateral pain symptoms immediately after the injury with these symptoms becoming more severe on the following day
- bilateral pain in serious cases, with the pain restricted to paravertebral muscles at the onset, then gradually involving the erector spinae, latissimus dorsi, trapezius and psoas major muscles
- in some cases, deviation or posterior protrusion of the spinous process and one or more tender points above the spinous ligaments
- inappropriate treatment at the acute stage will make the condition become chronic with climatic changes, prolonged sitting and standing, or bending of the waist. Patients with the chronic form of the condition often suffer distending back pain

TREATMENT
Acupoints and techniques

Combination of points	Needles used	Insertion technique	Needling sensation
Waiguan (SJ-5, bilateral)	No. 30 filiform needle, 1.5 cun in length	Insert perpendicularly to a depth of 0.5-1.0 cun towards Neiguan (PC-6)	Local distending pain or pain radiating to the middle finger
Local tender points: Three evident tender points beside the thoracic vertebral spinous process on the back	Three no. 30 filiform needles, 1.5 cun in length	Insert all three needles to a depth of 0.5-0.8 cun towards the spine	Local distending pain, which may radiate to the intercostal region on the same side or the anterior part of the thorax

Weizhong (BL-40, bilateral)	Two no. 30 filiform needles, 2 cun in length	Insert both needles perpendicularly to a depth of 1.0-1.2 cun	Regional distending pain

Method
- The patient adopts a sitting position.
- The acupoints are needled with the needles being retained for 40 minutes; during this period, one session of needle manipulation takes place.
- After the needles are withdrawn, cupping is performed immediately for one minute.
- Acupuncture should be performed once a day; one course of treatment consists of ten sessions.
- An interval of five days is required between two courses of treatment.

Clinical notes
Acupuncture is quite effective in treating this type of disorder. At the acute stage, three needling sessions bring relief to radiating pain in the thoracic intercostal spaces, respiratory pain and pain during coughing or sneezing. Pain of the neck and waist and local pain can be relieved after six to eight needling sessions. However, it is advisable to needle ten times to ensure no chronic symptoms remain.

This kind of treatment is also relatively satisfactory for treating chronic problems with frequent relapse, but the period of treatment required is longer. After recovery, the patient should be advised to increase exercise to prevent relapse.

11 INJURY TO THE ERECTOR SPINAE MUSCLE IN THE THORAX

Injury to the erector spinae muscle in the thorax is mainly associated with prolonged tension of the back and difficulty in relaxing the shoulders, the anterior part of the thorax and the back. It can arise in such instances as excessive strain caused by the carrying of heavy loads on the back or by teachers writing for long periods on the blackboard. This kind of excessive strain impairs the erector spinae muscle in the back and eventually causes pain.

Clinical manifestations
- chronic onset, frequently with unilateral involvement
- occurrence after thoracic movement, sleep or lifting a heavy object on one side
- pain usually begins from one side of the thoracic vertebrae with evident tenderness and gradually worsens
- intercostal pain
- for patients in serious pain, pain when breathing, coughing and sneezing
- limited movement of the scapula
- obvious tenderness on the back
- no obvious mass over the chest or scapular region

TREATMENT
Acupoints and techniques

Combination of points	Needles used	Insertion technique	Needling sensation
Tender points: Pain usually occurs beside the 3rd, 4th and 5th thoracic vertebrae; the three most evident tender points may be found beside these vertebrae	Three no. 30 filiform needles, 1.5 cun in length	Insert all three needles to a depth of 0.5-0.8 cun towards the spinal column	Local distending pain

Neiguan (PC-6, bilateral)	No. 30 filiform needle, 1.5 cun in length	Insert to a depth of 0.5-1.0 cun towards Waiguan (SJ-5)	Regional distending pain and/or pain radiating to the dorsum of the hand and middle finger

Method
- The patient lies in a prone position.
- The acupoints are needled with the needles being retained for 40 minutes; during this period, one session of needle manipulation takes place.
- After the needles are withdrawn, cupping therapy is performed immediately on the acupoints on the back for one minute.
- Acupuncture should be performed once a day; one course of treatment consists of six sessions.
- Treatment can recommence after an interval of three days, if necessary.

Clinical notes
Acupuncture appears to be effective in the treatment of injury to the erector spinae muscle in the thorax. The pain may be relieved after just six needling sessions. However, relapse frequently occurs, so patients are advised to undertake some not particularly strenuous forms of exercise, such as chest expanding, jogging or swimming. If a relapse does occur, the above methods may be reapplied.

12 INJURY TO THE PECTORALIS MAJOR MUSCLE

Presenting symptoms in the clinic mainly relate to injury to the origin or insertion of the pectoralis major muscle caused by direct or indirect force.

Injury is usually caused by overstrain of the upper arm or direct external trauma, such as may occur to workers involved in strenuous physical activities, athletes frequently using the upper limbs, or boxers. The symptoms may worsen under conditions of fatigue and cold weather.

Clinical manifestations
- evident history of trauma
- distending pain of the affected region over the chest, such as painful restriction of the origin or insertion of the pectoralis major muscle
- ecchymosis and distending pain over the affected region at the early stage; within one week, the pain gradually becomes worse, impairing the adduction of the upper arm (stretching the chest may worsen the pain) and the intercostal nerves, resulting in a radiating pain to the back
- involvement of the anterior part of the humerus below the shoulder or the part anterior to the armpit may result in the pain being exacerbated when abducting, extending or elevating the arm
- obvious tenderness or reflex pain over the impaired region

TREATMENT
Acupoints and techniques

Combination of points	Needles used	Insertion technique	Needling sensation
Bulang (KI-22, on the affected side)	No. 30 filiform needle, 1.5 cun in length	Insert to a depth of 0.5-0.8 cun slightly obliquely (at an angle of 15°) towards the sternum	Local distending pain
Shenfeng (KI-23, on the affected side)	No. 30 filiform needle, 1.5 cun in length	Insert to a depth of 0.5-0.8 cun slightly obliquely (at an angle of 15°) towards the sternum	Regional distending pain

Lingxu (KI-24, on the affected side)	No. 30 filiform needle, 1.5 cun in length	Insert to a depth of 0.5-0.8 cun slightly obliquely (at an angle of 15°) towards the sternum	Regional distending pain
Zhongfu (LU-1, on the affected side)	No. 30 filiform needle, 2 cun in length	Insert to a depth of 1.0-1.2 cun towards the shoulder joint	Regional distending pain
Neiguan (PC-6, on the affected side)	No. 30 filiform needle, 1.5 cun in length	Insert to a depth of 0.5-1.0 cun towards Waiguan (SJ-5)	Regional distending pain and/or pain radiating to the dorsum of the hand and middle finger

Method
- The patient lies in a supine position.
- The acupoints are needled with the needles being retained for 40 minutes; during this period, one session of needle manipulation takes place.
- After the needles are withdrawn, cupping therapy is performed on the needled acupoints for one minute.
- Acupuncture should be performed once a day; one course of treatment consists of six sessions.
- Treatment can recommence after an interval of three days if necessary.

Clinical notes
Acupuncture is effective in treating traumatic impairment and sprain of the pectoralis major muscle if no inflammation or damage to the periosteum is present, or if there is no fracture. The treatment is effective for most patients after one course. This method is also effective in treating damage to the periosteum after reduction of a fracture, but the treatment takes longer before it is effective.

13 COSTOCHONDRITIS (TIETZE'S SYNDROME)

Costochondritis is characterized by non-suppurative inflammation and the painful swelling of a rib (normally the second rib) resulting from swelling of the costochondral junctions.

The cause of the syndrome is unknown. However, it occurs most commonly when the costal cartilage is directly injured or crushed by such activities as stretching the chest or over-extending the arms during sports. The injury causes stagnation of regional Qi and blood and hinders the circulation of Qi and blood in the costal cartilage (according to TCM diagnosis).

Clinical manifestations
- often seen among young and middle-aged women
- commonly occurs at the costochondral junctions of the 2nd to 5th costal cartilages
- often seen unilaterally without any obvious history of preceding trauma
- in the early stages of the condition, there is evident distending pain that usually resolves in a week. Some cases gradually develop into chronic inflammation characterized by indistinct distension at the early stage, gradual worsening of pain and a firm immobile mass over the costal cartilage
- chest distress and referred pain below the affected shoulder may occur as well; in severe cases, there is coughing, heavy breathing and pain which worsens while stretching the chest and radiates to the back
- examination reveals a slight increase in the local skin temperature, palpable swelling on the affected costochondral joints and obvious tenderness

TREATMENT
Acupoints and techniques

Combination of points	Needles used	Insertion technique	Needling sensation
Location of obvious tender area on the affected side of the chest	Two no. 30 filiform needles, 1.5 cun in length	Insert laterally and slightly obliquely (at an angle of 15°) into the tender area for 0.5-0.8 cun	Regional distending pain

Neiguan (PC-6, on the affected side)	No. 30 filiform needle, 1.5 cun in length	Insert to a depth of 0.5-1.0 cun towards Waiguan (SJ-5)	Regional distending pain and/or pain radiating to the dorsum of the hand and middle finger
Yanglingquan (GB-34, on the affected side)	No. 30 filiform needle, 2 cun in length	Insert perpendicularly to a depth of 1.5 cun towards the interosseous membrane between the tibia and fibula	Regional distending pain

Method

- The patient lies in a supine position.
- The acupoints are needled with the needles being retained for 40 minutes; during this period, one session of needle manipulation takes place.
- After the needles are withdrawn, cupping therapy is performed on the chest for one minute.
- Acupuncture should be performed once a day; one course of treatment consists of six sessions.
- An interval of three days is required between two courses of treatment.

Clinical notes

At the early stage of the disorder, the swelling over the tender area is not obvious. It is painful on pressure and there is a slight discomfort in daily activities. Needling therapy is most effective at this stage. If the syndrome persists for a long period and there is obvious local pain and a large area of firm swelling with pain radiating to the shoulder and back, local corticosteroid injection is quite effective.

14 INJURY TO THE RECTUS ABDOMINIS MUSCLE

Pain in the abdomen due to over-contraction and torsion of the abdominal muscle is clinical evidence of an injury to the rectus abdominis muscle. This type of injury is often sustained by athletes such as runners or gymnasts specializing in parallel bars and the horizontal bar. Over-contraction during practice causes injury to the internal and external oblique muscles of the abdomen or an accumulation of acid substances in the muscles.

Clinical manifestations
- often seen among young and adult males
- obvious pain after sports with the pain involving the upper part of the rectus abdominis muscle below the costal arch or the middle part above the navel (the lower part is seldom involved)
- the pain usually occurs six hours after sporting activities. At the beginning there is only an uncomfortable sensation of the abdominal wall. The pain reaches a peak within about 24 hours and is characterized by an inability to walk
- in severe cases, the pain worsens when straightening the back, coughing, sneezing and rotating the trunk
- examination reveals no evident swelling of the abdomen, but tension of the rectus abdominis muscle and obvious tenderness below the costal arch or in the anterior sheath of the muscle above the navel

TREATMENT
Acupoints and techniques

Combination of points	Needles used	Insertion technique	Needling sensation
Zusanli (ST-36, bilateral)	Two no. 30 filiform needles, 2.5 cun in length	Insert perpendicularly to a depth of 1.8 cun	Regional distending pain or pain radiating to the dorsum of the foot

Abdominal tenderness: The most obvious tender area is located on both sides of the upper region of the abdomen or the navel. Usually the area of tenderness is large and is confined to the sheath of the rectus abdominis muscle	Four no. 30 filiform needles, 2 cun in length	Insert the first needle slightly obliquely (at an angle of 15°) into the tender area from its upper point to a depth of 1.5 cun; a second needle is inserted slightly obliquely (at an angle of 15°) above the navel to a depth of 1.5 cun. The insertion procedure is the same for both sides	Regional distending pain

Method

- The patient lies in a supine position.
- The acupoints are needled with the needles being retained for 40 minutes; during this period, one session of needle manipulation takes place.
- Cupping therapy is performed on the abdomen for one minute immediately after the needles are withdrawn.
- Acupuncture should be performed once a day; one course of treatment consists of six sessions.
- An interval of three days is required between two courses of treatment.

Clinical notes

This injury is rarely seen in the clinic and resolves without treatment within ten days in mild cases. Acupuncture treatment appears to be effective in treating the condition, which can be relieved after three sessions in mild cases and six sessions in severe ones. Patients are advised not to undertake strenuous sporting activities for one month after treatment to avoid recurrence of the injury.

15 SUPRASPINOUS LIGAMENT INJURY

Injury to the supraspinous ligament occurs as a result of prolonged physical work with bending of the waist, excessive physical exertion to move heavy objects or carrying heavy objects on the back, as well as from sudden events such as strenuous coughing or sneezing. These activities stretch the ligament, leading to oedema and possible laceration of the ligament. Unbearable pain occurs, spreading to the back.

Clinical manifestations
- occurs most frequently in young and adult males
- sudden onset even though torsional force was not necessarily strong; the 4th, 5th and 6th thoracic vertebrae are involved as well as the 3rd, 4th and 5th lumbar vertebrae
- the earliest symptom is pain in the spinous process of the affected thoracic and lumbar vertebrae, and in the interspinal muscle
- the pain worsens and the lower back stiffens the following day
- in severe cases, the pain is aggravated during coughing and sneezing, expanding upwards and downwards and developing from one to several spinous processes; it may also affect the interspinous ligaments and cause spasticity of the erector spinae
- the pain is worse when standing up, getting out of bed or bending
- patients usually walk with small steps and with their hands supporting the lower back region

TREATMENT
Acupoints and techniques

Combination of points	Needles used	Insertion technique	Needling sensation
Shuigou (DU-26)	No. 32 filiform needle, 1 cun in length	Insert obliquely upwards (at an angle of 45°) towards the upper maxilla to a depth of 0.3-0.5 cun	Regional distending pain

Tender areas: One or more tender areas can be found between the spinous processes on the back	No. 30 filiform needles, 1 cun in length (the number will vary according to the size of the tender area)	Insert obliquely upwards (at an angle of 45°) to a depth of 0.5-0.8 cun into the most obvious tender area along the space between the spinous processes	Regional distending pain
Weizhong (BL-40, bilateral)	Two no. 30 filiform needles, 2 cun in length	Insert perpendicularly to a depth of 1.0-1.2 cun	Regional distending pain

Method
- The patient lies in a prone position (the head should be turned to one side when locating DU-26).
- The acupoints are needled with the needles being retained for 40 minutes; during this period, one session of needle manipulation takes place.
- After the needles are withdrawn, cupping therapy is performed for one minute.
- Acupuncture should be performed once a day; one course of treatment consists of six sessions.
- An interval of three days is required between two courses of treatment.

Clinical notes
Acupuncture is effective in the treatment of injury to the supraspinous ligaments. The patient will experience relief after a course of six treatments.

16 PROLAPSE OF THE LUMBAR INTERVERTEBRAL DISC

The intervertebral disc suffers retrograde degeneration with advancing age, with dehydration of the nucleus pulposus and narrowing of the intervertebral space as well as laceration of the fibrous rings by trauma and impairment of the vertebral plate due to prolonged heavy physical work. Since the intervertebral disc often receives the heaviest pressure, it tends to protrude.

The fibrous rings of the intervertebral disc may become loose or lacerated, leading to the slow or sudden protrusion of the nucleus pulposus which then presses on the nerve root or spinal cord or both and results in various clinical symptoms.

Clinical manifestations

Clinically, the protrusion of the intervertebral disc can be divided into four categories.

Right protrusion:
- the nucleus pulposus protrudes to the right to cause compression of the root of the right spinal nerve
- pain is the main clinical symptom, radiating from the sciatic nerve to the lateral aspect of the shin and the dorsum of the foot
- there are three obvious locations of pain: the lower part of the buttock, the external side of the middle third of the thigh, and the lateral aspect of the shin
- there is one radiating pain point between the 4th and 5th lumbar vertebrae, or the 5th lumbar vertebra and 3 cm lateral to the median point of the 1st sacral vertebra on the affected side

Left protrusion:
- the nucleus pulposus protrudes to the left to cause compression of the root of left spinal nerve
- the clinical manifestations are the same as for the right protrusion

Central protrusion:
- the nucleus pulposus protrudes centrally to cause compression of the spinal cord
- the main clinical manifestations are numbness of the lower limbs and gradual occurrence of painful atrophy of the muscles; the pain worsens during sleep and is accompanied by aversion to cold

- pain and numbness worsen after movement. However, the pain is mild or moderate and not as serious as that of the lateral spinous process. The numbness is more serious and is aggravated when the vertebra is pressed

Mixed type:
- characterized by simultaneous right and central or left and central protrusion
- the main clinical manifestations are pain, numbness and atrophy of the muscles of the lower limb on the affected side along the path of the sciatic nerve, usually accompanied by migraine on the same side and backache
- pain and numbness are worse when pressure is put on the protruding part of the spinal column

Examination: X-ray examination is not routinely indicated and a "normal" plain X-ray may be falsely reassuring. MRI or CT scan may be undertaken if conservative management fails: the MRI scan is generally preferred and avoids irradiation.

TREATMENT
Acupoints and techniques

Combination of points	Needles used	Insertion technique	Needling sensation
Tender area: Located 1.0-1.5 cun lateral to the 4th and 5th lumbar vertebrae or the 5th lumbar vertebra and the 1st sacral vertebra	Two no. 26 filiform needles, 2.5 cun in length	The first needle is inserted perpendicularly in the tender area 1.0 cun from the spinal column to a depth of 1.5-2.0 cun towards the space of the spinous processes. The second needle is inserted perpendicularly in the tender area 1.5 cun from the spinal column to a depth of 1.5-2.0 cun towards the space of the transverse spinous processes	Distending pain radiating to the lower limbs and feet

Huantiao (GB-30, on the affected side or both sides)	No. 30 filiform needle, 3.5 cun in length	Insert to a depth of 2.5-3.0 cun towards the greater sciatic foramen	Regional distending pain or distending pain radiating to the sole
Zhibian (BL-54, on the affected side or both sides)	No. 30 filiform needle, 3 cun in length	Insert perpendicularly to a depth of 2.5 cun	Regional distending pain
Yinmen (BL-37, on the affected side or both sides)	No. 30 filiform needle, 2.5 cun in length	Insert perpendicularly to a depth of 2.0 cun	Regional distending pain
Weizhong (BL-40, on the affected side or both sides)	No. 30 filiform needle, 2 cun in length	Insert perpendicularly to a depth of 1.0-1.2 cun	Regional distending pain
Chengshan (BL-57, on the affected side or both sides)	No. 30 filiform needle, 2 cun in length	Insert perpendicularly to a depth of 1.5 cun	Regional distending pain

Method
- The patient lies in a prone position.
- The acupoints are needled on the affected side or both sides, with the needles being retained for 40 minutes; during this period, one session of needle manipulation takes place.
- After the needles are withdrawn, cupping therapy is performed for one minute.
- Acupuncture should be performed once a day; one course of treatment consists of ten sessions.
- An interval of five days is required between two courses of treatment.

Clinical notes
This therapy is quite effective in the treatment of small protrusions of the intervertebral disc (smaller than 0.5 cm). However, it is not so satisfactory in treating

large unilateral protrusions or mixed-type and central protrusions. Nevertheless, there is a certain effect in alleviating pain and relieving symptoms. If this therapy proves ineffective in clinical treatment, an operation should be considered to avoid delay in treatment and atrophy of the lower limbs. Acupuncture can reduce the pain and atrophy of the muscles after the operation. During the course of treatment or after the symptoms have been relieved, patients are advised to sleep on a very firm bed or place a board under their mattress. They should also exercise the lower limbs as much as possible, for example by walking backwards, to help the limbs recover their function.

17 INJURY TO THE ILIOPSOAS MUSCLE

The main clinical manifestations of this disorder are abdominal and lumbar pain as well as palsy of the femoral nerve.

The main causes of the injury are violent movement in such sports as gymnastics, hurdling or high jumping, or overloading of one side of the waist. The psoas major or iliacus muscle is injured or partially lacerated by violent contraction or excessive dragging of the iliopsoas muscle. The loose connective tissue between the aponeurosis of the iliopsoas muscle and the posterior peritoneum tends to lead to haematoma forming in the interstitial space in the loose connective tissue after damage to the iliopsoas muscle. This results in stimulation or pressure on the femoral nerve and leads to the clinical syndrome.

Clinical manifestations
- the patient has an obvious history of trauma
- early symptoms are distending pain of the iliopsoas, lumbar and abdominal regions, gradual aggravation accompanied by weakness of the quadriceps, numbness and constipation
- the patient tends to bend the waist
- external rotation of the thigh
- symptoms worsen during coughing and sneezing

Examination
- obvious haematoma in the lower abdomen and iliac fossa
- evident deep tenderness or pain radiating posteriorly to the waist under pressure; the pain appears in the groin, the anterior aspect of the thigh and the inner side of the leg under posterior pressure
- the iliac region cannot be straightened and the patient is lame
- positive iliofemoral nerve stretch test
- reduced or absent sensation at the front of the thigh and the femoral nerve distribution
- patellar tendon reflex reduced or absent
- the quadriceps muscle may be atrophied in patients suffering prolonged injury

TREATMENT
Acupoints and techniques

Combination of points	Needles used	Insertion technique	Needling sensation
Weidao (GB-28, on the affected side)	No. 30 filiform needle, 2 cun in length	Insert perpendicularly to a depth of 0.8-1.5 cun	Regional distending pain or pain radiating downwards along the front of the thigh
Fushe (SP-13, on the affected side)	No. 30 filiform needle, 1.5 cun in length	Insert perpendicularly to a depth of 1.0-1.2 cun	Regional distending pain
Biguan (ST-31, on the affected side)	No. 30 filiform needle, 2 cun in length	Insert perpendicularly to a depth of 1.5 cun	Regional distending pain
Xuehai (SP-10, on the affected side)	No. 30 filiform needle, 2 cun in length	Insert perpendicularly to a depth of 1.0-1.5 cun	Regional distending pain

Method
- The patient lies in a supine position.
- The acupoints are needled with the needles being retained for 40 minutes.
- After the needles are withdrawn, cupping therapy is performed for one minute.
- Acupuncture should be performed once a day; one course of treatment consists of ten sessions.
- An interval of five days is required between two courses of treatment.

Clinical notes
This therapy is effective three days after the injury has been sustained and should not be applied beforehand. Most patients can be cured after one course of treatment. However, a longer period is required to treat patients suffering prolonged injury accompanied by atrophy of the quadriceps or other muscles and palsy. The curative effect is also satisfactory in these cases. During the course of treatment, patients are advised to exercise the thigh muscles to promote earlier restoration of their function.

18 PAIN IN THE SACROCOCCYGEAL REGION

This syndrome is caused by degeneration of the coccygeal region or fracture of the coccyx.

The injury is often seen in patients who have fallen and landed on the base of the spine. It usually involves the sacrococcygeal joint and the coccygeal cartilage, manifesting as damage, fracture or dislocation of the involved part. It is difficult to treat and fixate the injured coccygeal vertebra, which often leads to anterior displacement of the distal part or abnormal union. In some women, the injury to the coccyx is caused by excessive abdominal pressure during childbirth. Stimulation and pressure on the injured sacrum may involve the peripheral tissues, tendons and coccygeal nerves, leading to acute or chronic pain. Prolonged sitting may press and rub the sacrococcygeal region, resulting in chronic injury of the sacrococcyx and leading to chronic pain.

Clinical manifestations
- most patients have a history of falling on the base of the spine or sustaining injury during childbirth
- pain usually occurs over the sacrococcygeal joint, manifesting as vague, dull or scorching pain
- in a few cases, pain may radiate to the perineum
- pain may worsen when sitting on a hard chair, defecating, coughing or sleeping for a prolonged period
- pain may also be induced by the alternating pressure of the buttocks when walking
- patients tend to raise the buttocks and bend the thigh to one side in the process of sitting down
- dry faeces and difficult defecation are usual symptoms

Examination: If patients have a history of abnormal union of sacrococcygeal fracture, examination of the anus reveals obvious tenderness and angulation of the coccyx.

TREATMENT
Acupoints and techniques

Combination of points	Needles used	Insertion technique	Needling sensation
Tender area: Obvious tenderness is often found in a radius 1 cm around Changqiang (DU-1)	Three no. 30 filiform needles, 1.5 cun in length	Insert the needles to a depth of 0.5-0.8 cun in the centre of the tender area towards the bone; insert one needle in the upper part of the area and two in the lower part (equidistant 1.5 cm from each other)	Regional distending pain
Weizhong (BL-40, bilateral)	Two no. 30 filiform needles, 2 cun in length	Insert perpendicularly to a depth of 1.0-1.2 cun	Regional distending pain

Method
- The patient lies in a prone position.
- The acupoints are needled with the needles being retained for 40 minutes; during this period, one session of needle manipulation takes place.
- After the needles are withdrawn, cupping therapy is performed for one minute.
- Acupuncture should be performed once a day; one course of treatment consists of six sessions.
- An interval of three days is required between two courses of treatment.

Clinical notes
Acupuncture is not used to treat sacrococcygeal bone syndrome at the acute stage of fracture. Pain caused by strain and childbirth can be treated satisfactorily by the above therapy. If patients do not respond after six treatments (one course), local corticosteroid injection could be considered. The curative effect is relatively satisfactory.
Note: After acupuncture and steroid injection treatment, some patients may experience a heavy distending sensation around the anus. This is a normal reaction.

19 SYNDROME OF THE THIRD LUMBAR TRANSVERSE PROCESS

Two main presentations are seen:
- Chronic overstrain: Prolonged work with the waist bent may result in injury due to chronic overstretching of the fulcrum, leading to multiple small muscular hernias and pain due to traction of the sensory branch of the lumbar nerve. This causes spasm of the regional muscles or chronic overstrain which subsequently leads to oedema, exudation and fibrous hyperplasia around the transverse process of the lumbar vertebra or synovitis of the articular process.
- Sprain due to sudden bending of the waist: Laceration of the tendons around the lumbar vertebrae can lead to inflammation or muscular hernia.

Clinical manifestations
- chronic unilateral or bilateral pain of the lower back
- aggravation of pain when getting out of bed or bending the waist
- difficulty in straightening the lower back, attenuation of pain after completion of movement, continuous pain in most cases
- radiation of pain from the buttocks to the lateral side of the thigh or the lateral side of the knee in a few cases
- examination reveals normal movement of the lumbar vertebrae, obvious tenderness around the transverse process of the 3rd lumbar vertebra, hard nodules and fibrous soft tissue palpable in some cases, and numbness or sensitive regions around the 2nd and 3rd lumbar vertebrae or sacral region.

TREATMENT
Acupoints and techniques

Combination of points	Needles used	Insertion technique	Needling sensation
Shenshu (BL-23, bilateral)	Four no. 30 filiform needles, 2 cun in length	Insert the first needle obliquely to a depth of 1.0-1.5 cun, the second is inserted obliquely 0.5 cun below the first one to a depth of 1.0-1.5 cun (both sides)	Local distending pain

Weizhong (BL-40, bilateral)	Two no. 30 filiform needles, 2 cun in length	Insert perpendicularly to a depth of 1.0-1.2 cun	Regional distending pain

Method
- The patient lies in a prone position.
- The acupoints are needled with the needles being retained for 40 minutes; during this period, one session of needle manipulation takes place.
- After the needles are withdrawn, cupping therapy is performed for one minute.
- Acupuncture should be performed once a day; one course of treatment consists of six sessions.
- An interval of three days is required between two courses of treatment.

Clinical notes
This syndrome is common. Most cases can be treated satisfactorily by needling, but needling is ineffective for a few patients because of the length of the illness and stubborn pathology. In these instances, local corticosteroid injection can be considered.

20 SNAPPING HIP

This condition often occurs when the hip joint is flexed or stretched and is commonly seen among young people.

Normally the movement of the hip joint does not cause pain and snapping. However, when certain factors cause the hip joint and surrounding muscles to loosen, friction of the upper part of the trochanter and the acetabulum may result in snapping when the hip joint stretches or flexes. Generally, this condition does not affect movement of the hip joint and causes no pain. However, prolonged snapping may cause pain due to erosion of the facet of the acetabulum.

Clinical manifestations
- in the early stages, snapping of the hip joint only occurs during movement. A clear snapping can be heard in flexion
- at the advanced stage, snapping is often accompanied by pain

TREATMENT
Acupoints and techniques

Combination of points	Needles used	Insertion technique	Needling sensation
Tender area (on the affected side): Obvious tenderness often appears below or above Huantiao (GB-30)	No. 28 filiform needle, 3.5 cun in length	Insert perpendicularly to a depth of 2.5-3.0 cun into the tender area	Distending pain in the hip joint
Jiaji 17th (EX-B-2, on the affected side)	No. 30 filiform needle, 1.5 cun in length	Insert perpendicularly to a depth of 0.5-1.0 cun	Regional distending pain or pain radiating to the hip
Zhibian (BL-54, on the affected side)	No. 28 filiform needle, 3 cun in length	Insert perpendicularly to a depth of 2.5 cun	Regional distending pain
Weizhong (BL-40, on the affected side)	No. 30 filiform needle, 2 cun in length	Insert perpendicularly to a depth of 1.0-1.2 cun	Regional distending pain

Method
- The patient lies on the non-affected side.
- The acupoints are needled with the needles being retained for 40 minutes; during this period, one session of needle manipulation takes place.
- After the needles are withdrawn, cupping therapy is performed for one minute.
- Acupuncture should be performed once a day; one course of treatment consists of ten sessions.
- An interval of five days is required between two courses of treatment.

Clinical notes
Snapping without pain is often overlooked. In some cases, the problem resolves spontaneously. However, obvious snapping accompanied by pain should be treated by this therapy, which has proved effective. After recovering, patients are advised to exercise more or take up a sport to prevent snapping of the hip joint.

21 LUMBOSACRAL LIPOCOELE

This condition is often seen among obese middle-aged and elderly women. It results from the accumulation of lumbosacral fat that progressively distends the lumbosacral fascia and vascular foramen and loosens them. Under certain situations, fat may protrude to cause compression, stimulation and traction of local tissues.

Clinical manifestations
- unilateral occurrence is often seen among women aged 30 to 40, while bilateral occurrence is commonly found among people in the 45 to 60 age range
- there is no traumatic history or premonitory signs
- the condition usually occurs with pain after fatigue; the pain appears continuous
- in some cases, the pain is related to climatic changes and is reduced after rest
- when the lipocoele occurs at the level of the 4th to 5th lumbar vertebrae and deep in the posterior crest of the ilium, the pain radiates to the popliteal fossa. The pain is usually dull rather than sharp
- above the sacral region, the lipocoele is often found 2 cun lateral to the 2nd and 3rd sacral vertebrae. Large lipocoeles that persist for a long time can stimulate and pull the sciatic nerve, leading to slight sciatica

Examination
- one or more smooth nodules (the size of a chestnut or walnut) can be found over one or both crests behind the ilium
- the nodules are characterized by a hard core and an elastic body. They can be pushed aside within a certain range but immediately return to the original position. Distending pain is felt when pressed

TREATMENT
Acupoints and techniques

Combination of points	Needles used	Insertion technique	Needling sensation
Tender area: Obvious tenderness or nodules can be found in the lumbar or sacral region	In the lumbar region, two no. 28 filiform needles, 3 cun in length are used for each point; in the sacral region, two no. 30 filiform needles, 2 cun in length, are used for each point	In the lumbar region, insert perpendicularly to a depth of 2.0 cun at a point situated respectively above and below the tender or nodule area at a distance of about one-third of the diameter of the area; in the sacral region, insert perpendicularly to a depth of 1.5 cun at similar points	Regional distending pain or pain radiating to the lower limb
Weizhong (BL-40, on the affected side or both sides)	No. 30 filiform needle, 2 cun in length	Insert perpendicularly to a depth of 1.0-1.2 cun	Regional distending pain

Method
- The patient lies in a prone position.
- The acupoints are needled with the needles being retained for 40 minutes; during this period, one session of needle manipulation takes place.
- After the needles are withdrawn, cupping therapy is performed for one minute.
- Acupuncture should be performed once a day; one course of treatment consists of six sessions.
- An interval of three days is required between two courses of treatment.

Clinical notes
Lumbosacral lipocoele responds well to this therapy. Usually pain can be alleviated or relieved in six sessions. In some mild cases, the nodules disappear after needling. Where there are large nodules, they gradually soften during the treatment and the pain gradually diminishes. Recurrence is likely.

22 LUMBAR SPONDYLOSIS

Lumbar spondylosis is characterized by degenerative hyperplasia of the vertebral margins and the joint cartilage.

Its cause is not clear, although some researchers believe that degeneration of the vertebral body and surrounding tissues plays a major role. Common manifestations are degeneration of the intervertebral disc, collapse of the vertebral body, narrowing of the intervertebral disc space, bony lipping of the vertebral body and spinous hyperplasia, and hyperplasia of the intervertebral small joints. However, hyperplasia does not necessarily lead to clinical symptoms. This problem has also been related to obesity and endocrine disorders.

Clinical manifestations
- often occurs in middle-aged people
- some patients have an obvious history of trauma before the onset of the disease
- in most cases, onset is slow. Clinically, it is related to the location of the hyperplasia, such as pathological changes in the 1st, 2nd and 3rd lumbar vertebrae
- if onset is slow and the 3rd, 4th and 5th lumbar vertebrae are involved, the pain usually starts from the waist and gradually develops to the affected side or both popliteal fossae
- in acute cases, onset in one day may cause sciatica on the same side, leading to pain of the lower limbs along the distribution of the sciatic nerve. The pain becomes serious at night; it is relieved after movement and aggravated with a stiff back and backache after strenuous activity

Examination
- obvious tenderness may be found beside the lumbar spinous process
- X-ray examination indicates osteophytic lipping of vertebrae at multiple levels, sometimes with bony fusion, as well as narrowing of the intervertebral space

TREATMENT
Acupoints and techniques

Combination of points	Needles used	Insertion technique	Needling sensation
Shenshu (BL-23, bilateral)	Two no. 30 filiform needles, 2 cun in length	Insert obliquely to a depth of 1.0-1.5 cun	Regional distending pain or pain radiating to the lower limb on the same side
Dachangshu (BL-25, bilateral)	Two no. 30 filiform needles, 2 cun in length	Insert perpendicularly to a depth of 1.5 cun	Regional distending pain or pain radiating to the lower limb and sole
Weizhong (BL-40, bilateral)	Two no. 30 filiform needles, 2 cun in length	Insert perpendicularly to a depth of 1.0-1.2 cun	Regional distending pain

Method
- This therapy is applicable to lumbar spondylosis with chronic onset and lumbar pain.
- The patient lies in a prone position.
- The acupoints are needled with the needles being retained for 40 minutes; during this period, one session of needle manipulation takes place.
- After the needles are withdrawn, cupping therapy is performed for one minute.
- Acupuncture should be performed once a day; one course of treatment consists of ten sessions.
- An interval of five days is required between two courses of treatment.

Clinical notes
Lumbar spondylosis is commonly seen. It can be treated effectively by this therapy, but there is a marked tendency to relapse. Patients are advised to undertake some form of physical activity after the pain disappears, for example by exercising the lower back or walking backwards. Relapse can also be treated effectively by the above therapy.

23 **SYNOVIAL BURSITIS OF THE HIP**

This is a pathological change of the hip characterized by pain in the hip and impaired hip movement and is commonly encountered.

Synovial bursitis is caused by a variety of factors, such as tuberculosis and rheumatism. It may also be caused by chronic abduction and external rotation of the lower limb, such as when jumping or doing the splits, and by over-fatigue (which distorts or squeezes the bursa) followed by an attack of wind-cold (according to TCM diagnosis).

Clinical manifestations
- such symptoms as swelling, pain and difficulty in walking are obvious after acute sprain of the hip joint
- some patients only feel discomfort of the joint region immediately after the injury and can walk normally. However, pain is aggravated in the next few days, eventually appearing while walking and standing; this pain may make the patients limp
- patients tend to incline their pelvis to one side to alleviate the pain
- in some patients, low fever appears due to local blood stasis (according to TCM diagnosis)

Examination
- no obvious tenderness in the hip joint region, but pain can be induced by standing, walking, flexion and adduction
- in some patients, swelling or mild tenderness appears in the area of the greater trochanter

TREATMENT
Acupoints and techniques

Combination of points	Needles used	Insertion technique	Needling sensation
Zhibian (BL-54, on the affected side)	No. 30 filiform needle, 3 cun in length	Insert to a depth of 2.5 cun towards the hip joint	Regional distending pain or pain radiating to the lower limb and sole

Chengfu (BL-36, on the affected side)	No. 30 filiform needle, 2.5 cun in length	Insert perpendicularly to a depth of 2.0 cun	Regional distending pain
Dachangshu (BL-25, on the affected side)	No. 30 filiform needle, 3 cun in length	Insert to a depth of 2.5 cun towards the space of the transverse processes of the 4th and 5th lumbar vertebrae	Regional distending pain or pain radiating to the lower limb
Tender area (on the affected side): Usually tenderness in movement appears on the median point of the line connecting the tuberosity on the greater femoral trochanter and Huantiao (GB-30)	No. 26 filiform needle, 3 cun in length	Insert 2.5 cun towards the hip joint capsule	Regional distending pain

Method
- The patient lies on the non-affected side.
- The acupoints are needled with the needles being retained for 40 minutes; during this period, one session of needle manipulation takes place.
- After the needles are withdrawn, cupping therapy is performed for one minute.
- Acupuncture should be performed once a day; one course of treatment consists of ten sessions.
- An interval of five days is required between two courses of treatment.

Clinical notes
Using filiform needles to treat this disease is relatively effective in stopping the pain. However, needling alone is not completely effective in treating adhesions as a result of the chronic inflammation around the hip joint, which should be treated by needling combined with local corticosteroid injection.

24 INJURY TO THE SACROSPINALIS MUSCLE IN THE LUMBAR REGION

This injury is mainly caused by prolonged sitting, and affects such people as drivers, teachers and office workers. Prolonged sitting leads to chronic sprain or acute injury to the sacrospinalis muscle as a result of continual tension of the muscle. Improper treatment will turn the sprain into chronic injury.

Clinical manifestations
- patients often have a history of acute sprain or trauma
- onset is sudden, usually occurring when getting out of bed or where the patient adopts an improper lower back position
- pain is sharp and appears mainly in the lower back in the initial stage. Inappropriate treatment in the first two days may cause the pain to spread to the lower limbs
- in most cases, the pain only radiates to the popliteal region of the affected side; there is not usually any pain in the shin
- in serious cases, the pain is aggravated when lying down, standing up, turning the body, or coughing and sneezing
- there is obvious tenderness beside the 3rd and 4th lumbar vertebrae, but the pain does not radiate to the lower limbs under pressure

TREATMENT
Acupoints and techniques

Combination of points	Needles used	Insertion technique	Needling sensation
Qihaishu (BL-24, on the affected side or both sides)	No. 30 filiform needle, 2 cun in length	Insert perpendicularly to a depth of 1.5 cun	Regional distending pain or pain radiating to the ipsilateral lower limb
Dachangshu (BL-25, on the affected side or both sides)	No. 30 filiform needle, 2 cun in length	Insert perpendicularly to a depth of 1.5 cun	Regional distending pain or pain radiating to the lower limb and sole

Weizhong (BL-40, on the affected side or both sides)	No. 30 filiform needle, 2 cun in length	Insert perpendicularly to a depth of 1.0-1.2 cun	Regional distending pain

Method
- The patient lies in a prone position.
- The acupoints are needled with the needles being retained for 40 minutes; during this period, one session of needle manipulation takes place.
- After the needles are withdrawn, cupping therapy is performed for one minute.
- Acupuncture should be performed once a day; one course of treatment consists of six sessions.
- An interval of three days is required between two courses of treatment.

Clinical notes
Early treatment of this injury is very effective. In most cases, pain can be relieved after four or five needling sessions. Patients suffering from this injury for a prolonged period can also be satisfactorily treated by this therapy, but a longer course of treatment is required. After recovery, patients are advised to undertake more sporting activities to strengthen the power of their lumbar muscles so as to prevent relapse.

25 ACUTE SPRAIN OF THE LOWER BACK

The main symptom of this condition is acute lumbar pain due to sudden sprain of the lumbar soft tissues or excessive stretching.

Sprain is usually caused by indirect external force, such as excessive posterior extension, flexion, rotation or bending of the waist and is commonly seen among labourers due to improper posture. In some cases, patients do not undertake sufficient physical exercise, so the inclination of the lower back may cause acute sprain of the lumbar muscles.

Clinical manifestations
- often occurs among the middle-aged and elderly who have an obvious history of trauma
- in most cases, pain appears when a "clicking" sound is heard during sprain of the lower back
- pain is usually unilateral, rarely bilateral
- most patients feel pain immediately after the sprain, being unable to move or bend at the waist
- pain is worse when sitting down, coughing, sneezing, taking a deep breath or walking
- some patients may only feel distending discomfort of the lower back at the onset but experience great pain after one or two days; in these cases, pain is milder initially and can only be felt when standing up or sitting down
- pain worsens when patients bend at the waist or make an effort to do something, but is absent when breathing and coughing

Examination: One or more tender areas can be found at the 3rd, 4th and 5th lumbar vertebrae on the affected side. In some patients, an elongated mass can be felt.

TREATMENT
Acupoints and techniques

Combination of points	Needles used	Insertion technique	Needling sensation
Shenshu (BL-23, on the affected side)	No. 30 filiform needle, 2 cun in length	Insert obliquely to a depth of 1.0-1.5 cun	Regional distending pain or pain radiating to the ipsilateral lower limb
Qihaishu (BL-24, on the affected side)	No. 30 filiform needle, 2 cun in length	Insert perpendicularly to a depth of 1.5 cun	Regional distending pain or pain radiating to the ipsilateral lower limb
Yinmen (BL-37, on the affected side)	No. 30 filiform needle, 2.5 cun in length	Insert perpendicularly to a depth of 2.0 cun	Regional distending pain
Weizhong (BL-40, on the affected side)	No. 30 filiform needle, 2 cun in length	Insert perpendicularly to a depth of 1.0-1.2 cun	Regional distending pain
Yaotongdian (EX-UE-7, bilateral)	Four no. 30 filiform needles, 1.5 cun in length	Insert obliquely upwards (at an angle of 45°) to a depth of 1.0 cun	Local distending pain

Method
- The patient lies in a prone position.
- With the exception of EX-UE-7, the acupoints are needled with the needles being retained for 40 minutes; during this period, one session of needle manipulation takes place.
- After the needles are withdrawn, cupping therapy is performed for one minute.
- The technique is a little different at EX-UE-7, where the needles are manipulated with larger amplitude for two minutes after insertion. During

manipulation, patients are asked to move their waist slowly or to move it in the direction of the pain. The needles are retained for 30 minutes and are manipulated once more when they are withdrawn. The needling technique is the same on both sides.

• Acupuncture should be performed once a day until full recovery.

Clinical notes

EX-UE-7 alone can be needled for cases treated within 48 hours of onset. Some patients can be cured after just one treatment session. If the pain cannot be relieved, then the four body acupoints can be applied the next day. If EX-UE-7 is ineffective in the treatment of conditions older than two days, only the four body acupoints should be chosen.

Clinically, acute sprain of the lower back is one of the commonly encountered forms of lumbago. In some cases, it appears as habitual sprain of the lower back. Frequent attacks, even those brought about by coughing and sneezing, can be treated effectively by needling. Recently-afflicted patients can be given relief by needling EX-UE-7 once only. Two further sessions of body needling can completely relieve the pain. Where patients have been afflicted for longer, six needling sessions can usually provide basic relief of the pain if needling is accurate. After recovery, patients are advised to undertake some form of jogging or running to strengthen their body to avoid habitual sprain of the lower back.

Chapter 3

Upper limb conditions

26 SEQUELAE OF SCAPULAR FRACTURE

This is a syndrome caused by prolonged irritation of local tissues from adhesions caused by repair of a fracture of the body, neck, spine, coracoid process or acromion of the scapula.

Clinical manifestations
- the main symptoms are pain and restriction of movement affecting the top of the shoulder and the supraspinatus and infraspinatus muscles
- if the fracture occurs in the acromion or coracoid process, the pain usually extends over the upper part of the shoulder and is aggravated when the upper arm is abducted
- if the fracture is depressed or fragments of the bone have damaged the adjacent nerves, numbness of the upper limb may be felt
- injury to the radial nerve may be encountered
- at a later stage, the pain in the supraspinatus and infraspinatus muscles is often exacerbated when the neck is extended and suffers pressure during sleep; obvious tenderness is usually found in the shoulder or back in these cases
- X-ray examination indicates previous fracture of the scapula

TREATMENT
Acupoints and techniques

Combination of points	Needles used	Insertion technique	Needling sensation
Tender area: One or more tender areas can be found above the shoulder or over the supraspinatus and infraspinatus muscles. The number of filiform needles used depends on the size of the tender area	No. 30 filiform needles, 2 cun in length	See below	Distending pain over the shoulder and supraspinatus and infraspinatus muscles
Quchi (LI-11, on the affected side)	No. 30 filiform needle, 2 cun in length	Insert perpendicularly to a depth of 1.2-1.5 cun	Regional distending pain

Hegu (LI-4, on the affected side)	No. 30 filiform needle, 2 cun in length	Insert to a depth of 1.0-1.5 cun towards Houxi (SI-3)	Regional distending pain

Insertion technique: Within the tender area on the shoulder, one needle is inserted to a depth of 1.0 cun towards the shoulder joint near the bone. Within the tender area of the supraspinatus muscle, one needle is inserted to a depth of 0.5-0.8 cun along the muscle into the supraspinous fossa. Two or three needles may be inserted horizontally to puncture larger areas of tenderness. To puncture the infraspinatus muscle, the needle is inserted to a depth of 1.0-1.2 cun along the muscle into the infraspinous fossa. If the tender area is located around Jianjing (GB-21), horizontal needling to a depth of 0.5 cun is used to avoid damage to the pleura or lung.

Method
- The patient adopts a sitting position.
- Electro-acupuncture is performed on the acupoints; the stimulation must be monitored to remain within the tolerance level of the patient.
- The needles are retained for 40 minutes. After the needles are withdrawn, cupping therapy is performed for one minute.
- Treatment is applied once a day; one course consists of ten treatments.
- An interval of five days is required between two courses of treatment.

Clinical notes
If patients have local pain and restriction of arm movement, a longer course of treatment is required. However, the curative effect is also satisfactory. During the treatment, patients should be advised to increase shoulder movements to promote earlier recovery.

27 SUBACROMIAL BURSITIS

This condition results from inflammation of the subacromial bursa due to overstrain. Inappropriate treatment will lead to thickening of the wall of the bursa and adhesion formation. These changes result in the failure of the buffering function of the bursa, affecting extension, elevation and rotation of the shoulder joint and causing pain during movement. This problem often exists along with chronic inflammation of soft tissue.

Clinical manifestations
- distending pain of the affected shoulder is an early clinical symptom
- there may be no obvious tender area; the pain is aggravated when the shoulder is elevated, abducted or when carrying a load
- at the later stage, an effusion may occur, causing exacerbation of pain during the night; there is an obvious tender area and swelling below the acromion, and severe pain occurs when the shoulder is moved
- if the effusion continues to increase, a swelling can be found posterior and anterior to the shoulder joint
- when the condition is severe, pain may radiate to the upper arm and neck

TREATMENT
Acupoints and techniques

Combination of points	Needles used	Insertion technique	Needling sensation
Taijian point (on the affected side): Located in the depression below the acromio-clavicular joint (see diagram, page 167)	No. 28 filiform needle, 2 cun in length	Insert perpendicularly towards the shoulder joint to a depth of 1.2-1.5 cun	Regional distending pain
Jianyu (LI-15, on the affected side)	No. 30 filiform needle, 2 cun in length	Insert to a depth of 1.5 cun towards the elbow along the long axis of the humerus	Regional distending pain or pain radiating to the elbow

Naoshu (SI-10, on the affected side)	No. 28 filiform needle, 2 cun in length	Insert perpendicularly to a depth of 1.5 cun towards the front of the shoulder	Regional distending pain
Quchi (LI-11, on the affected side)	No. 30 filiform needle, 2 cun in length	Insert for 1.2-1.5 cun towards Shaohai (HT-3) in the subcutaneous plane	Regional distending pain

Method
- The patient adopts a sitting position.
- The forearm should be rested on a flat surface with the medial aspect parallel to the body so that LI-11 and HT-3 are in vertical alignment.
- The acupoints are needled with the needles being retained for 40 minutes; during this period, one session of needle manipulation takes place.
- After the needles are withdrawn, cupping therapy is performed for one minute.
- Treatment is applied once a day; one course consists of ten treatments.
- An interval of five days is required between two courses of treatment.

Clinical notes
Needling therapy is effective in treating subacromial bursitis in the absence of effusion. Corticosteroid injection is more effective in treating the condition when there is an effusion. A longer course of treatment is required to treat serious adhesion due to local inflammation, which should be treated by corticosteroid injection followed by ordinary needling, or by needling combined with electro-acupuncture. During convalescence, patients should be advised to perform shoulder exercises, for example rotational movements. Needling may also be done in combination with massage to relax local adhesions. Treatment with these therapies is usually effective.

28 SEQUELAE OF CLAVICULAR FRACTURE

Clavicular fracture is a common injury. Various local symptoms are produced by damage to the local tissues and vessels after fracture, or by tension of the muscles around the shoulder and clavicle while the fracture is mending.

Clinical manifestations
- obvious history of clavicular fracture
- the main symptom is pain of the upper arm during movement
- the tender areas are usually located anterior to the shoulder and below the sternoclavicular joint
- pain is aggravated when the upper arm is elevated or abducted to a horizontal level or carries heavy objects
- asymmetry between the affected shoulder joints and the sternoclavicular joint
- X-ray examination indicates previous fracture of the clavicle

TREATMENT
Acupoints and techniques

Combination of points	Needles used	Insertion technique	Needling sensation
Tender area: Obvious tenderness can be found at the superior or inferior borders of the acromioclavicular joint and the inferior border of the sternoclavicular joint	No. 28 filiform needle, 1 cun in length	Insert from the tender area towards the joint to a depth of 0.5 cun	Regional distending pain
Lanwei (EX-LE-7, on the affected side)	No. 30 filiform needle, 2 cun in length	Insert perpendicularly to a depth of 1.5 cun	Regional distending pain or pain radiating to the dorsum of the foot

Method

- The patient adopts a sitting position.
- The acupoints are needled with the needles being retained for 40 minutes; during this period, one session of needle manipulation takes place. Electro-acupuncture can be used to needle the acupoints on the shoulder.
- After the needles are withdrawn, cupping therapy can be performed for one minute.
- Treatment is applied once a day; one course consists of ten treatments.
- An interval of five days is required between two courses of treatment.

Clinical notes

Sequelae of clavicular fracture are commonly encountered. The above therapy is very effective in treating this stubborn condition. To treat patients with local adhesions, needling should be followed by electro-acupuncture. During treatment or after the pain has been relieved, patients should exercise their upper arm to help relieve adhesions and avoid relapse.

29 SUPRASPINATUS TENDINITIS

This condition is often seen among young and middle-aged people, most of whom have a history of trauma. It is caused by a variety of factors, such as carrying loads, sprain, contusion or minor trauma, all of which may lead to chronic inflammation of the tendon of the supraspinatus muscle.

Clinical manifestations
- usually occurs on the dominant side
- symptoms are often not obvious in the beginning, frequently little more than a distending pain over the supraspinatus muscle and aggravation of pain during shoulder abduction
- as the condition develops, the symptoms gradually worsen, leading to restricted active abduction of the shoulder. The pain is often restricted to the part above the spine of the scapula or the back of the shoulder, radiating to the upper part of the arm and the elbow, and to the trapezius muscle

Examination
- tenderness is found on the greater tuberosity of the humerus or the origin of the deltoid muscle
- obvious pain is caused when abduction is in the range of 60°-100°; the pain disappears when the abduction exceeds 120°, because the muscle is free from the friction of the acromion, but the pain is felt again when the elbow is lowered: clinically, this is known as painful arc syndrome
- X-ray examination may show calcification of the supraspinatus tendon

TREATMENT
Acupoints and techniques

Combination of points	Needles used	Insertion technique	Needling sensation
Tender area: Obvious tenderness can be found over the acromion (near the origin of the deltoid muscle)	No. 28 filiform needle, 2.5 cun in length	Insert in the centre of the tender area to a depth of 1.5 cun towards the shoulder joint	Regional distending pain

Jianjing (GB-21, on the affected side)	No. 30 filiform needle, 1.5 cun in length	Insert obliquely (at an angle of 45°) to a depth of 1.0 cun towards the spine of the scapula. Horizontal needling is used to avoid damage to the pleura or lung	Regional distending pain
Jianzhongshu (SI-15, on the affected side)	No. 30 filiform needle, 1.5 cun in length	Insert obliquely (at an angle of 45°) to a depth of 1.0 cun towards the spinal column	Regional distending pain
Quchi (LI-11, on the affected side)	No. 30 filiform needle, 2 cun in length	Insert perpendicularly to a depth of 1.2-1.5 cun	Regional distending pain

Method
- The patient lies in a supine position.
- The acupoints are needled with the needles being retained for 40 minutes; during this period, one session of needle manipulation takes place.
- After the needles are withdrawn, cupping therapy is performed for one minute.
- Treatment is applied once a day; one course consists of six treatments.
- An interval of three days is required between two courses of treatment.

Clinical notes
This therapy is relatively effective in treating supraspinatus tendinitis. Corticosteroid injection is only used when the condition has persisted for a long period and needling is not particularly effective. It is better to use acupuncture treatment at an early stage, because one or two days after corticosteroid injection the pain is aggravated due to absorption of the drugs. Patients should be forewarned of this.

30 TENDINITIS OF THE FOREARM EXTENSOR MUSCLES

Tendinitis of the forearm extensor muscles is caused by aseptic inflammation of the tendons due to a variety of injuries.

Injury to the long and short extensor tendons of the thumb is commonly encountered. It often develops in people working in such trades as carpentry, construction and shipbuilding.

Clinical manifestations
- often seen among young and middle-aged people with a history of obvious pain
- the painful area is characterized by swelling, warmth of the overlying skin, obvious tenderness, aggravation when the thumb, index and middle fingers are extended against resistance and when the wrist is extended; the symptoms are alleviated by rest
- when the problem is prolonged, it leads to local chronic inflammation and adhesions, affecting flexion and extension of the fingers and wrist

Examination
- obvious swelling, tenderness, and an increase in skin temperature usually found on the radial side superior to the wrist (approximately corresponding to Lieque [LU-7])
- pain is aggravated when the thumb and wrist are extended

TREATMENT
Acupoints and techniques

Combination of points	Needles used	Insertion technique	Needling sensation
Tender area: The most obvious tenderness on the prominence can be found on the radial side of the area above the wrist on the affected side (corresponding to Lieque [LU-7])	Two no. 30 filiform needles, 1.5 cun in length	Insert to a depth of 0.5 cun towards the ulna with 1.0 cun between the two acupoints at the tender area	Regional distending pain

Quchi (LI-11, on the affected side)	No. 30 filiform needle, 2 cun in length	Insert for 1.2-1.5 cun towards Shaohai (HT-3) in the subcutaneous plane	Regional distending pain
Hegu (LI-4, on the affected side)	No. 30 filiform needle, 2 cun in length	Insert to a depth of 1.0-1.5 cun towards Houxi (SI-3)	Regional distending pain

Method
- The patient adopts a sitting position.
- The forearm should be rested on a flat surface with the medial aspect parallel to the body so that LI-11 and HT-3 are in vertical alignment.
- The acupoints are needled with the needles being retained for 40 minutes; during this period, one session of needle manipulation is carried out.
- After the needles are withdrawn, cupping therapy is performed for one minute.
- Treatment is applied once a day; one course consists of six treatments.
- An interval of three days is required between two courses of treatment.

Clinical notes
This therapy is relatively effective in treating the disorder in the acute phase, requiring three to five days of treatment for a cure. Inappropriate treatment may lead to adhesion of the tendons, which will require a longer period of therapy. However, this can also be treated satisfactorily by careful use of this method.

31 SUPINATOR SYNDROME

Supinator syndrome is caused by pressure on the radial nerve due to injury to the supinator muscle and other factors.

Pressure on the radial nerve may be caused by stimulation and traumatic degenerative inflammation, deformity of the tuberosity of the radius, thickening of the interosseous membrane during development, abnormal union of the upper third of the radius, and stubborn lateral epicondylitis of the humerus.

Clinical manifestations
- dorsal interosseous nerve pressure is commonly seen
- the main symptoms are obvious restriction of extension of the thumb and metacarpophalangeal joints
- obvious referred pain felt if the metacarpal joints are extended
- the other obvious symptom is impaired function of the supinator, but there is no sensory disturbance

Examination
- obvious painful nodules can be felt in the area around Shousanli (LI-10)
- pain worsens during supination and pronation of the forearm
- electromyography: abnormal electric potentials may appear in some patients

TREATMENT
Acupoints and techniques

Combination of points	Needles used	Insertion technique	Needling sensation
Shousanli (LI-10, on the affected side)	No. 30 filiform needle, 2 cun in length	Insert perpendicularly to a depth of 1.5 cun	Distending pain radiating to the dorsum of the hand or the middle finger
Quchi (LI-11, on the affected side)	No. 30 filiform needle, 2 cun in length	Insert for 1.2-1.5 cun towards Shaohai (HT-3) in the subcutaneous plane	Regional distending pain

Shouwuli (LI-13, on the affected side)	No. 30 filiform needle, 1 cun in length	Insert perpendicularly to a depth of 0.5-0.8 cun	Local distending pain or pain radiating to the radial side of the wrist
Waiguan (SJ-5, on the affected side)	No. 30 filiform needle, 1.5 cun in length	Insert perpendicularly to a depth of 0.5-1.0 cun towards Neiguan (PC-6)	Local distending pain or pain radiating to the middle finger

Method

- The patient adopts a sitting position.
- The forearm should be rested on a flat surface with the medial aspect parallel to the body so that LI-11 and HT-3 are in vertical alignment.
- The acupoints are needled with the needles being retained for 40 minutes; during this period, one session of needle manipulation is carried out.
- After the needles are withdrawn, cupping therapy is performed for one minute.
- Treatment is applied once a day; one course consists of ten treatments.
- An interval of five days is required between two courses of treatment.

Clinical notes

Supinator syndrome can be effectively treated by needling, but other disorders must be excluded. If there is larger local swelling (an elongated mass due to spasm of local muscles or sclerosis of the tendons), electro-acupuncture can be used. During and after the treatment, patients should be advised to avoid carrying anything heavy or forcefully supinating the affected forearm, in order to avoid relapse.

32 OLECRANON BURSITIS

This condition can be classified into acute and chronic forms. A heavy jolt may cause acute bursitis, for example from falling, when a goalkeeper dives to the ground or when a wrestler falls and hits the ground with his elbow. This type of injury may cause bleeding into the bursa and swelling, leading to the acute condition. Excessive violent flexion of the elbow as in gymnastics, throwing the javelin or weightlifting may damage the bursa. Chronic olecranon bursitis may be caused by prolonged friction of the elbow against the ground, for example when miners or soldiers are crawling using the elbows.

Clinical manifestations
- in acute cases, a history of trauma is the main characteristic causing immediate swelling, pain, tenderness and fluctuation of the bursa as well as mild restriction of elbow movement
- the injury should be differentiated from haematoma due to contusion of the back of the elbow and rupture of the tendon of the triceps muscle. With contusion of the elbow, the haematoma is small and usually extends to the distal end of the dorsal side of the ulna with subcutaneous ecchymosis. In cases of rupture of the tendon of the triceps muscle, there is a depression over the rupture
- chronic olecranon bursitis occurs gradually and is often discovered by accident after several injuries. The non-tender swelling is usually round or oblong and varies in size; it is located below the olecranon. The firmness of the swelling is associated with thickness of the bursal wall and an effusion. If there is calcification, the swelling is usually hard and movement of the elbow is slightly restricted

Examination
- obvious tenderness, an increase in skin temperature and a fluctuant mass between the olecranon and the lateral humeral epicondyle. If the bursitis is prolonged, there may be restriction of elbow movements and muscle atrophy
- X-ray examination may show calcification of the bursa in some patients

TREATMENT
Acupoints and techniques

Combination of points	Needles used	Insertion technique	Needling sensation
Sidu (SJ-9, on the affected side)	No. 30 filiform needle, 2 cun in length	Insert perpendicularly to a depth of 1.0-1.5 cun	Regional distending pain or pain radiating to the middle finger
Tianjing (SJ-10, on the affected side)	No. 30 filiform needle, 1.5 cun in length	Insert to a depth of 1.3 cun into the ligament between the lateral humeral epicondyle and the olecranon	Regional distending pain or pain radiating to the fourth and fifth fingers
Qinglengyuan (SJ-11, on the affected side)	No. 30 filiform needle, 2 cun in length	Insert obliquely upwards (at an angle of 45°) to a depth of 1.5 cun	Distending pain radiating to the shoulder or to the radial side of the wrist

Method
- The patient adopts a sitting position.
- The acupoints are needled with the needles being retained for 40 minutes; during this period, one session of needle manipulation is carried out.
- After the needles are withdrawn, cupping therapy is performed for one minute.
- Treatment is applied once a day; one course consists of six treatments.
- An interval of three days is required between two courses of treatment.

Clinical notes
Needling is effective in treating olecranon bursitis, both at the early stage where there is no significant effusion, or where it is chronic. If there is adhesion or calcification, electro-acupuncture should be used. If there is significant effusion, corticosteroid injection is the most effective treatment.

33 LATERAL HUMERAL EPICONDYLITIS (TENNIS ELBOW)

The causes of this condition are not fully understood. Repeated, prolonged and violent overexertion of the elbow and wrist occurring as a result of playing tennis, injury to the elbow joint, or twisting something with great force appear to be the main factors. Relapse is frequent. In some cases, local symptoms develop above and below the epicondyle. Other names may be used for this condition, such as general tendinitis, fibrositis or epicondylitis. Prolonged chronic inflammation may also cause oedema of granulation tissue, with organization of haemorrhage and dense adhesions, eventually resulting in degeneration of the tissues.

Clinical manifestations
- onset is gradual and slow in most cases; undue exertion may cause sudden onset and gradual aggravation with pain
- at the early stage, the pain is dull or continuous
- the condition may improve or disappear in two or three months if there are no aggravating factors
- in cases of frequent recurrence, the pain does not disappear spontaneously; instead it becomes worse and is aggravated by such activities as twisting a towel, picking up a cup, cleaning the floor, fastening buttons, or flexing or pronating the forearm
- at an advanced stage, the pain radiates above and below the epicondyle, involving the tendons of the wrist extensors and the tendon of extensor carpi radialis, leading to stiffness of the elbow and problems of wrist extension

Examination
- obvious tenderness and swelling over the lateral humeral condyle
- wrist extension against resistance causes pain
- X-ray examination is not routinely indicated, but may show calcification, periosteal reaction and roughness of the lateral humeral condyle at the advanced stage

TREATMENT
Acupoints and techniques

Combination of points	Needles used	Insertion technique	Needling sensation
Tender area (on the affected side): Obvious tenderness can be found on the lateral humeral epicondyle	No. 30 filiform needle, 1 cun in length	Insert to a depth of 0.5 cun slightly downwards towards the radial surface	Regional distending pain or pain radiating to the radial side of the arm
Shouwuli (LI-13, on the affected side)	No. 30 filiform needle, 1 cun in length	Insert perpendicularly to a depth of 0.5-0.8 cun	Local distending pain or pain radiating to the radial side of the wrist
Shousanli (LI-10, on the affected side)	No. 30 filiform needle, 2 cun in length	Insert perpendicularly to a depth of 1.5 cun	Distending pain radiating to the dorsum of the hand or the middle finger

Method
- The patient adopts a sitting position.
- The acupoints are needled with the needles being retained for 40 minutes; during this period, one session of needle manipulation is carried out.
- After the needles are withdrawn, cupping therapy is performed for one minute.
- Treatment is applied once a day; one course consists of six treatments.
- An interval of three days is required between two courses of treatment.

Clinical notes
Tennis elbow can be effectively treated by needling at an early stage. However, needling therapy is not so effective for treatment at the intermediate or advanced stages, where it can be satisfactorily treated by local corticosteroid injection. Sharp pain will be experienced one day after steroid injection as the drugs are absorbed. Relapse is frequent with this type of condition. Patients are therefore advised to avoid any activities that may cause relapse, such as playing tennis, or wrenching or twisting the wrist.

34 MEDIAL HUMERAL EPICONDYLITIS (GOLFER'S ELBOW)

Local inflammation is caused by repeated tension, contraction, flexion and overstrain of the flexor muscles of the forearm. Damage to the pectoralis major muscle may also lead to tension and contraction of the muscles of the forearm.

Clinical manifestations
- distending pain on the ulnar side below the elbow on the affected side
- pressure on the ulnar nerve may ensue, leading to such symptoms as intermittent numb pain of the fourth and fifth fingers which may disturb sleep, as well as distending pain radiating above and below the medial epicondyle in advanced cases

Examination
- obvious tender area at the medial humeral epicondyle, wrist flexion against resistance causes pain
- X-ray examination is not routinely indicated but may show periosteal reaction around the medial humeral epicondyle

TREATMENT
Acupoints and techniques

Combination of points	Needles used	Insertion technique	Needling sensation
Shaohai (HT-3, on the affected side)	No. 30 filiform needle, 1 cun in length	Insert to a depth of 0.3-0.5 cun towards Quchi (LI-11)	Regional distending pain or pain radiating to the external side of the little finger
Qingling (HT-2, on the affected side)	No. 30 filiform needle, 2 cun in length	Insert perpendicularly, then move horizontally proximally 1.5 cun along the medial side of the humerus against the bone	Transmitted upwards towards the armpit or scapula

Tender area (on the affected side): Tenderness is found superior to the medial epicondyle on the affected side	No. 30 filiform needle, 1 cun in length	Insert to a depth of 0.5 cun towards the ulna against the bone	Regional distending pain or pain transmitted to the small thenar eminence

Method
- The patient adopts a sitting position.
- The acupoints are needled with the needles being retained for 40 minutes; during this period, one session of needle manipulation is carried out.
- After the needles are withdrawn, cupping therapy is performed for one minute.
- Treatment is applied once a day; one course consists of six treatments.
- If this treatment is ineffective, local corticosteroid injection can be used.

Clinical notes
Golfer's elbow can be treated effectively by needling therapy. However, it may also be necessary to use corticosteroid injection to treat patients with a chronic condition, when frequent relapse occurs, or where acupuncture has not achieved a satisfactory effect. To treat patients with prolonged sleep disturbance, corticosteroid injection can be performed on Shenmen (HT-7). The efficacy is satisfactory. Relapse can also be effectively treated by this therapy.

35 BICIPITAL TENDINITIS

This condition is usually caused by repeated movements and strain, causing pain at the origin of the biceps muscle.

Bicipital tendinitis often occurs among labourers doing physical work over a long period. Frequent trauma, sprain or contusion maintains inflammation in the local region, causing congestion, exudation and swelling as well as changes in the synovial sheath surrounding the tendon. This leads to degeneration of the tissues. The disorder often occurs together with rotator cuff impingement.

Clinical manifestations
- usually occurs among the young and middle-aged
- protective spasm of the deltoid muscle often appears at the acute stage
- local tumescent pain and evident tenderness can be felt at the coracoid process at the origin of the short head of the biceps
- symptoms are exacerbated during movement and alleviated after rest

Examination
- obvious tenderness at the coracoid process
- flexing the elbow against resistance causes pain
- during contraction of the biceps, crepitus can be felt in the tender area, which is localized to the bicipital groove
- frozen shoulder may occur

TREATMENT
Acupoints and techniques

Combination of points	Needles used	Insertion technique	Needling sensation
Tender area: Obvious tenderness or crepitant sensation can be located on the coracoid process anterior to the inferior part of the acromion	Two no. 28 filiform needles, 2 cun in length	Insert perpendicularly to a depth of 1.5 cun on the superior and inferior sides of the tender area	Local distending pain
Lanwei (EX-LE-7, on the affected side)	No. 30 filiform needle, 2 cun in length	Insert perpendicularly to a depth of 1.5 cun	Local distending pain or pain radiating to the dorsum of the foot

Tianfu (LU-3, on the affected side)	No. 30 filiform needle, 2 cun in length	The biceps muscle is lifted slightly and the needle is inserted perpendicularly to a depth of 1.5-1.8 cun through the tendons and aponeurosis inferior to the biceps muscle	Local distending pain or pain radiating to the elbow

Method

- The patient adopts a sitting position.
- The needle is first inserted into EX-LE-7 and manipulated by the fingers with large amplitude and at high frequency. At the same time, the patient is asked to move the shoulder as much as possible. Needle manipulation and patient movement should continue until the pain is alleviated. Then the other three needles are inserted (the patient must remain still when the needles are inserted into the shoulder).
- The needles are retained for 40 minutes, during which time one session of needle manipulation is carried out.
- After the needles are withdrawn, cupping therapy is performed on the shoulder for one minute.
- Treatment is applied once daily on alternate days; one course consists of six treatments.
- If one course does not prove effective, the treatment should be stopped.

Clinical notes

Acupuncture treatment of this disorder is extremely effective if undertaken at the early stage. However, although acupuncture is helpful in treating the disease at an advanced stage or in helping patients with frozen shoulder or tendinitis around the shoulder, its results are not totally satisfactory. Under these conditions, the needling or corticosteroid injection therapies detailed in sections 36 or 29 can be employed. If local adhesions are obvious, routine treatment may be carried out in combination with electro-acupuncture, which has proven to be an effective method.

36 **FROZEN SHOULDER (SCAPULOHUMERAL PERIARTHRITIS)**

This is a complicated syndrome, often seen among people over 50 years of age (more frequently in women than men). It may be caused by prolonged overstrain, sprain, contusion or exposure of the shoulder during sleep, leading to chronic inflammation of the tissues and nerve fibres around the shoulder. In the early stages, mild pain or tenderness may occur at the front of the shoulder, below the tip of the acromion or at the back of the shoulder. As the condition gradually develops, it leads to such symptoms as restricted movement of the shoulder joint, pain which worsens at night, and tenderness at several places around the shoulder. At an advanced stage, the manifestations are a lower degree of pain, obvious tenderness on pressure, restricted movement of the shoulder, with adhesions, calcification and stiffness of the capsular tissues as well as various degrees of atrophy of the muscles around the shoulder.

Clinical manifestations
Clinically, the condition is divided into three stages:
Early stage:
- no obvious pain, one or more tender areas may be found on the shoulder
- the function of the shoulder is not restricted; pain may sometimes be felt for a short period during movement
- there may be a leucocytosis in some patients

Intermediate stage:
- pain or sharp tenderness, worse at night
- obvious local swelling
- pain worsens when the shoulder is moved
- increase in local skin temperature and restricted movement of the shoulder
- there may be a leucocytosis in some patients

Advanced stage:
- the shoulder is stiff and movement causes pain
- pain occurs at night and one or more nodules appear on the shoulder
- restriction of such activities as dressing and undressing, and combing the hair
- the muscles around the shoulder become atrophic
- X-rays may indicate calcification in some patients

TREATMENT
Acupoints and techniques

Combination of points	Needles used	Insertion technique	Needling sensation
Lanwei (EX-LE-7, on the affected side)	No. 30 filiform needle, 2 cun in length	Insert perpendicularly to a depth of 1.5 cun	Regional distending pain or pain radiating to the dorsum of the foot
Taijian point (on the affected side): Located in the depression below the acromio-clavicular joint (see diagram, page 167)	No. 28 filiform needle, 1.5 cun in length	Insert perpendicularly to a depth of 1.0-1.2 cun towards the back of the shoulder	Regional distending pain
Jianyu (LI-15, on the affected side)	No. 28 filiform needle, 2 cun in length	Insert to a depth of 1.8 cun towards the shoulder joint along the space between the greater and lesser tuberosities of the humerus	Regional distending pain or pain radiating to the upper part of the elbow
Naoshu (SI-10, on the affected side)	No. 28 filiform needle, 2 cun in length	Insert perpendicularly to a depth of 1.5 cun towards the front of the shoulder	Regional distending pain

Method
- The patient adopts a sitting position.
- The acupoints are needled with the needles being retained for 40 minutes; during this period, one session of needle manipulation takes place.
- After the needles are withdrawn, cupping therapy is performed for one minute.
- Treatment is applied once a day; one course consists of ten treatments.
- An interval of five days is required between two courses of treatment.

Clinical notes

EX-LE-7 alone can be needled to treat frozen shoulder at the early stage. In this case, the needle should be manipulated strongly on insertion; at the same time, patients should move the affected shoulder as much as possible until it can be raised somewhat and the pain alleviated. The needle is retained for 40 minutes. When the needle is about to be withdrawn, it should again be manipulated strongly to strengthen stimulation. Sometimes, two or three needling sessions are sufficient to effect a complete cure.

To treat patients at the intermediate stage, this method is used in combination with the three acupoints located on the shoulders. Needling therapy is not quite so effective in treating patients at the advanced stage, where treatment by electro-acupuncture, corticosteroid injection to the tender area, exercises and massage are required. Nevertheless, generally speaking, needling therapy is a satisfactory treatment for frozen shoulder.

37 SEQUELAE OF OLECRANON FRACTURE

These sequelae refer to the symptoms which become apparent after treatment of a fracture of the olecranon, such as local pain, adhesions and restricted movement of the elbow joint.

This condition arises mainly as a result of direct trauma, such as falling onto the olecranon, or from an indirect force such as falling on the outstretched hand or excessive twisting of the elbow joint during a throwing action. Fractures can be classified into comminuted fracture, avulsion fracture, and greenstick fracture.

The sequelae of olecranon fracture can be divided into two categories:

a) Restriction of both flexion and extension:

These are sequelae of conservative treatment (such as plaster fixation or splint) of comminuted or greenstick fractures. The main cause is injury to the tissues, the tendons and the vessels in the joint cavity of the elbow during fracture of the olecranon. This results in such symptoms as rupture of the small blood vessels, fibrous tissues or synovial cavity, bruising of the tissues or an elbow joint effusion.

b) Restriction of flexion:

These symptoms are caused by comminuted fracture of the olecranon, avulsion fracture, injury during the repair or operative removal of comminuted fragments, or abnormal union of the fracture.

Clinical manifestations
Restriction of both flexion and extension
- the forearm and upper arm are in a flexion position of 130°-160°
- obvious tenderness and oedema at the point where the biceps muscle is inserted into the olecranon; oedema appears at the radial side below the elbow joint
- painful restriction of the elbow joint when extended; the biceps muscle shows obvious protective spasm when the elbow is extended

Restriction of flexion
- the elbow retains a position of rigid extension
- scar left after operation or nodular substance left after abnormal union of the wound near the olecranon and the triceps muscle; one or more tender areas are found at the olecranon

TREATMENT
Acupoints and techniques

Combination of points	Needles used	Insertion technique	Needling sensation
Quchi (LI-11, on the affected side)	No. 30 filiform needle, 2 cun in length	Insert for 1.2-1.5 cun towards HT-3 in the subcutaneous plane	Regional distending pain
Shaohai (HT-3, on the affected side)	No. 30 filiform needle, 1 cun in length	Insert to a depth of 0.3-0.5 cun towards LI-11	Regional distending pain or pain radiating to the external side of the little finger
Tianjing (SJ-10, on the affected side)	No. 28 filiform needle, 1.5 cun in length	Insert to a depth of 1.0 cun towards the olecranon	Regional distending pain
Tender area: When the elbow is flexed, a very obvious tender area is located between Sidu (SJ-9) and Tianjing (SJ-10) and also between the radius and the ulna (see diagram, page 163)	No. 30 filiform needle, 2 cun in length	Insert to a depth of 1.5 cun towards PC-3	Regional distending pain or pain radiating to the middle finger
Area on the tendon below the biceps muscle (on the affected side): When the elbow flexes and the biceps muscle contracts slightly, the area below the prominence of the muscle is selected for needling (see diagram, page 166)	No. 30 filiform needle, 2 cun in length	Insert to a depth of 1.5 cun towards the humerus	Regional distending pain

Quze (PC-3, on the affected side)	No. 30 filiform needle, 2 cun in length	Insert to a depth of 0.8-1.0 cun towards the humerus	Regional distending pain

Method

Restriction of both flexion and extension

- The patient adopts a sitting position.
- The main needling point is HT-3, which is combined with PC-3 and SJ-10 and the area between SJ-9 and SJ-10.
- The acupoints are needled as described above in combination with electro-acupuncture monitored to ensure it remains within the patient's tolerance level.
- The needles are retained for 40 minutes.
- After the needles are withdrawn, cupping therapy is performed for one minute.

Restriction of flexion

- The patient adopts a sitting position.
- The main acupoint selected is the tender area between SJ-9 and SJ-10, combined with LI-11, HT-3 and the area on the tendon below the biceps muscle. These acupoints are needled in combination with electro-acupuncture monitored to ensure it remains within the patient's tolerance level.
- The needles are retained for 40 minutes.
- After the needles are withdrawn, cupping therapy is performed for one minute.

- Both therapies are applied once a day; one course consists of ten treatments.
- An interval of five days is required between two courses of treatment.

Clinical notes

Electro-acupuncture should be used at an early stage. This method is especially effective in relieving adhesions when treating patients with restriction of both flexion and extension. If the therapy described above is insufficient to relieve the restriction of flexion, it should be combined with functional exercises to increase effectiveness.

38 ULNAR NERVE COMPRESSION

This syndrome is caused by pressure on the ulnar nerve at the wrist. It has two main causes:
- Local pressure: direct pressure on the ulnar nerve by problems within the confined space as the nerve passes over the flexor retinaculum, such as ganglion, angioma or lipoma.
- Thickening of the flexor retinaculum: trauma and repeated injury, especially chronic professional injury, result in fibrous degeneration, thickening and scar formation of the retinaculum. This leads to a reduction in the volume of the canal and pressure on the ulnar nerve.

Clinical manifestations
- the syndrome varies according to the location and degree of pressure on the ulnar nerve
- pressure of the deep branch of the ulnar nerve may cause weakness, atrophy and numbness; pressure on the ulnar nerve canal at the wrist may involve the superficial branch of the ulnar nerve, resulting in pain and weakness over the region of ulnar nerve distribution
- movement of the wrist on the affected side usually induces such symptoms as aggravated pain during the night, which sometimes radiates to the elbow or appears intermittently in some patients

Examination
- typical clawed deformity of the fingers and atrophy of the intrinsic muscles and hypothenar eminence resulting in weak finger abduction and thumb adduction: pinching is difficult
- sensation is diminished or lost over the little finger and the ulnar border of the ring finger
- pressure on the internal border of the pisiform bone and the medial side of the ulna may worsen the symptoms

TREATMENT
Acupoints and techniques

Combination of points	Needles used	Insertion technique	Needling sensation
Shenmen (HT-7, on the affected side)	No. 30 filiform needle, 1 cun in length	Insert to a depth of 0.3-0.5 cun towards Yangxi (LI-5)	Regional distending pain or pain radiating to the tip of the little finger
Houxi (SI-3, on the affected side)	No. 30 filiform needle, 2 cun in length	Insert to a depth of 1.8 cun towards Hegu (LI-4)	Regional distending pain
Zhongzhu (SJ-3, on the affected side)	No. 30 filiform needle, 1.5 cun in length	Insert to a depth of 0.5-0.8 cun towards the pisiform bone	Regional distending pain or pain radiating to the tip of the little finger
Shaohai (HT-3, on the affected side)	No. 30 filiform needle, 1 cun in length	Insert to a depth of 0.3-0.5 cun towards Quchi (LI-11)	Regional distending pain or pain radiating to the external side of the little finger

Method
- The patient adopts a sitting position.
- The acupoints are needled with the needles being retained for 40 minutes.
- Treatment is applied once a day; one course consists of ten treatments.
- An interval of five days is required between two courses of treatment.

Clinical notes
Electro-acupuncture is the most effective treatment of this condition at the early stage. A longer course of treatment is necessary in dealing with cases at an advanced stage, but the curative effect is satisfactory. During the course of treatment, patients are advised to avoid coming into contact with cold objects so as not to diminish the curative effect.

39 STENOSING TENOSYNOVITIS (DE QUERVAIN'S DISEASE)

This painful condition, which mainly affects women, is caused by chronic sprain of the wrist.

Overstraining the wrist in such activities as regular packing of boxes, sewing, carrying children or loading and unloading may cause excessive inflammation and thickening of the sheath containing the tendons of extensor pollicis brevis and the abductor pollicis longus. If the condition persists, it may result in oedema, thickening of the tendon wall, swelling and roughness of the tendon, and excessive secretion of synovial fluid, leading to distending pain.

Clinical manifestations
- commonly seen among middle-aged and elderly women and younger women 2-3 months after childbirth
- in the acute stage, obvious local distension or pain in the depression at the styloid process of the radius
- increased local skin temperature and aggravation of pain on abduction of the thumb; in serious cases, the pain may radiate to the elbow

Examination
- obvious tender area at the tip of the radial styloid process
- there may be swelling along the course of the thumb tendons

TREATMENT
Acupoints and techniques

Combination of points	Needles used	Insertion technique	Needling sensation
Yangxi (LI-5, on the affected side)	No. 30 filiform needle, 1 cun in length	Insert to a depth of 0.3 cun into the depression of the bone	Regional distending pain or pain radiating to the dorsal side of the thumb
Hegu (LI-4, on the affected side)	No. 30 filiform needle, 1.5 cun in length	Insert obliquely upwards (at an angle of 45°) to a depth of 1.0 cun	Regional distending pain

Shousanli (LI-10, on the affected side)	No. 30 filiform needle, 2 cun in length	Insert perpendicularly to a depth of 1.5 cun	Distending pain radiating to the dorsum of the hand or the middle finger

Method
- The patient adopts a sitting position.
- The acupoints are needled with the needles being retained for 40 minutes; during this period, one session of needle manipulation is carried out.
- Treatment is applied once a day; one course consists of six treatments.
- If ineffective, corticosteroid injection may be considered.

Clinical notes
Acupuncture is very effective in the treatment of this problem at an early stage. If the pain is so serious that the thumb cannot be abducted, corticosteroid injection into the tendon sheath should be considered; the curative effect is satisfactory. However, the administration of the corticosteroid injection should be carefully controlled. This condition tends to relapse. After recovery, patients should therefore be advised to avoid excessive use of the wrist. Relapse can be effectively treated by the therapies described above.

40 CARPAL TUNNEL SYNDROME

This syndrome is commonest in menopausal women but can also be associated with pregnancy or rheumatoid arthritis. Occasionally it may be caused by injury to the wrist and pressure on the median nerve, abnormal union of a carpal fracture, dislocation of the lunate bone, carpal tunnel abscess and pressure on the carpal canal from a ganglion or lipoma. The main manifestations are aseptic inflammation and oedema of the tissues in the carpal tunnel resulting in pressure and stimulation on the median nerve.

Clinical manifestations
- numbness of the thumb, index and middle fingers and the radial border of the ring finger
- wasting of the thenar eminence
- in serious cases, evident impairment of the functions of the thumb, index and middle fingers in grasping objects
- pain is aggravated during sleep and after fatigue and cold stimulation; alleviation of pain is felt after slight movement or application of a hot compress
- hanging the arm over the side of the bed or shaking the hand may relieve symptoms
- pain may radiate to the elbow and shoulder in some cases

Examination
- there may be tenderness in the carpal canal
- some flaccidity or atrophy of the thenar eminence
- hypoaesthesia of the thumb, index and middle fingers and the ulnar border of the ring finger
- X-ray examination may show arthritis, stenosis of the carpal tunnel or old fracture or dislocation of the lunate bone
- nerve conduction studies may show decreased conduction velocity in the median nerve

TREATMENT
Acupoints and techniques

Combination of points	Needles used	Insertion technique	Needling sensation
Daling (PC-7, on the affected side)	No. 30 filiform needle, 1 cun in length	Insert perpendicularly to a depth of 0.3-0.5 cun	Regional distending pain or pain radiating to the index and middle fingers
Hegu (LI-4, on the affected side)	No. 30 filiform needle, 2 cun in length	Insert to a depth of 1.0-1.5 cun towards Houxi (SI-3)	Regional distending pain
Neiguan (PC-6, on the affected side)	No. 30 filiform needle, 1.5 cun in length	Insert towards Waiguan (SJ-5) to a depth of 0.5-1.0 cun	Regional distending pain and/or pain radiating to the dorsum of the hand and middle finger

Method
- The patient adopts a sitting position.
- The acupoints are needled with the needles being retained for 40 minutes; during this period, one session of needle manipulation is carried out.
- After the needle is withdrawn, cupping therapy is performed for one minute on PC-7.
- Treatment is applied once a day; one course consists of six treatments.
- An interval of three days is required between two courses of treatment.

Clinical notes
At the early stage, needling achieves satisfactory treatment of symptoms characterized by local distending pain and a slight, numb distension of the thumb, index and middle fingers. However, with such symptoms as aggravated pain at night, numbness of the finger tips and restriction of the digital functions, needling alone is not fully effective. Corticosteroid injection can then be used to relieve pain, followed by needling and electro-acupuncture to deal with atrophy of the muscles. The treatment chosen should depend on the underlying cause.

41 INJURY TO THE TRIANGULAR CARTILAGE

This injury is caused by the rotation, friction, pulling or fracture dislocation of the distal part of the radius. Wrist pain is the main symptom.

Clinical manifestations
- obvious history of trauma
- evident swelling and tenderness at the junction of the lunate and triquetral bones
- reduced power of grasping, with failure to hold objects firmly
- if the condition becomes chronic, pain is aggravated by extension and supination/pronation of the wrist, possibly with snapping of the wrist joint

Examination
- obvious tenderness over the dorsum of the wrist between Yangchi (SJ-4) and Yanggu (SI-5)
- restriction of rotation of the carpal joint
- flattening of the depression below the ulna
- pressure test on the triangular cartilage disk evokes pain

TREATMENT
Acupoints and techniques

Combination of points	Needles used	Insertion technique	Needling sensation
Yanglao (SI-6, on the affected side)	No. 30 filiform needle, 1 cun in length	Insert perpendicularly to a depth of 0.3-0.5 cun	Regional distending pain
Yanggu (SI-5, on the affected side)	No. 30 filiform needle, 1 cun in length	Insert to a depth of 0.3-0.5 cun towards the interosseous space (see clinical notes below)	Regional distending pain

Sidu (SJ-9, on the affected side)	No. 30 filiform needle, 2 cun in length	Insert perpendicularly to a depth of 1.0-1.5 cun	Regional distending pain or pain radiating to the middle finger
Zhongzhu (SJ-3, on the affected side)	No. 30 filiform needle, 1 cun in length	Insert to a depth of 0.5 cun towards SJ-4	Regional distending pain

Method
- The patient adopts a sitting position.
- The acupoints are needled with the needles being retained for 40 minutes; during this period, one session of needle manipulation is carried out.
- Treatment is applied once a day; one course consists of six treatments.
- An interval of three days is required between two courses of treatment.

Clinical notes
Acupuncture has proved effective in treating the pain caused by this condition and can restore the functions of the wrist. In needling SI-5, the needle is inserted perpendicularly into the interosseous space. The pain this causes is so great that some patients cannot bear it. Those who can tolerate the pain will certainly benefit. If the condition is accompanied by impaired wrist function, electro-acupuncture is effective.

42 TENOVAGINITIS OF THE DIGITAL FLEXOR MUSCLES

This condition is caused by inflammation of the tendons of the digital flexor muscles.

Clinical manifestations
- often occurs among women and is associated with overstrain (such as spinning and weaving, packing and sewing). It is sometimes congenital and may only be discovered at the age of 12-18 months when the thumb cannot flex
- often involves the thumb, middle and fourth fingers
- prolonged overstrain of the finger joints results in sprain and friction of the tendons of the deep and superficial flexor muscles causing injury to the fibrous sheath surrounding the tendons, chronic aseptic inflammation and eventually oedema, degeneration or calcification of the cartilage, stenosis and adhesions of the sheath, with thickening of the tendon
- snapping and pain can be felt when the tendons of the deep and superficial flexor muscles move within the narrowed sheath during flexion and extension
- the main early symptoms include painful restriction of flexion of the wrist and fingers, with weakness in grasping objects
- a gradually enlarging elongated firm swelling appears in the sheath in the palm
- in serious cases, entrapment is frequent and pain is aggravated on passively relieving the flexor muscles, and there is rigidity of the joints beyond the affected area
- examination: obvious tender area in the tendon sheath of the flexor muscles in the palm

TREATMENT
Acupoints and techniques

Combination of points	Needles used	Insertion technique	Needling sensation
Tender area (on the affected side): The most obvious tender area or nodular mass is located on the affected palm	No. 30 filiform needle, 1.5 cun in length	Insert perpendicularly to a depth of 0.5-0.8 cun towards the metacarpophalangeal joint	Regional distending pain

Daling (PC-7, on the affected side)	No. 28 filiform needle, 2 cun in length	Insert into the skin and then move horizontally towards the tender area. If other tendon sheaths become painful, more needles are inserted into the tender area	Regional distending pain

Method
- The patient adopts a sitting position.
- The acupoints are needled with the needles being retained for 40 minutes; during this period, one session of needle manipulation is carried out.
- Treatment is applied once every other day; one course consists of six treatments.
- Stop the treatment if it is ineffective after one course.

Clinical notes
Acupuncture is relatively effective in treating the pain caused by this syndrome. However, a complete cure depends mainly on corticosteroid injection. Two hours after administering the injection, pain will gradually worsen as a normal reaction to drug absorption. Patients should be told to expect this. The pain will generally disappear after 24 hours. If the patient is not cured after one or two treatments, corticosteroid injections should be halted. This condition has a tendency to relapse.

43 WRITER'S CRAMP

Writer's cramp is a functional impairment of writing characterized by spasmodic contraction and abnormal movement of the muscles of the hand and forearm.

The pathogenesis of the disease is not clear. The patient can function normally in daily life without impaired muscle function. However, examination performed when the patient exhibits symptoms may show increased muscle tone of the finger and wrist muscles and resistance can be felt when the wrist joint is passively pronated or supinated. In a few patients, the thumb is held in an abnormal position of lateral rotation, and some individuals show lack of co-ordination of arm movements when walking.

Clinical manifestations

- the most characteristic feature of the disease is spasm during writing; when the patient is not writing, the symptom disappears and muscular tone is completely normal
- sometimes the writing difficulty only occurs when a pen is used and the patient writes completely normally with a pencil

Clinically, the disease can be divided into three types:

Spasmodic type (hypermyotonic type):
- the most common type; muscular spasm occurs shortly after writing begins
- the index finger extends fully, whereas the thumb and other fingers are flexed
- the interosseous, forearm and shoulder muscles contract shortly thereafter and this is accompanied by severe pain

Paralytic type (hypomyotonic type):
- when writing, the patient cannot use a pen, feels tired, asthenic and incapable of voluntary movement because of flaccid muscle tone; sometimes there is pain along the nerve pathway

Tremor type (hyperkinetic type):
- when writing, a tremor develops, especially under emotional influence

TREATMENT
Acupoints and techniques

Combination of points	Needles used	Insertion technique	Needling sensation
Praxis area (on the healthy side): Defined by three 3 cm lines, the central line extending from the parietal tuberosity to the centre of the mastoid process, and the other two anterior and posterior to the central line with an angle of 40° between them (see diagram, page 165)	Three no. 30 filiform needles, 1.5 cun in length	Starting from the central point of the parietal tuberosity, three horizontal punctures are made, one inferiorly, and one anteriorly and one posteriorly at an angle of 20° to the first one, each to a depth of about 1.2 cm	Local distending pain
Hegu (LI-4, on the affected side)	No. 30 filiform needle, 2 cun in length	Insert towards Yuji (LU-10) for about 1.6 cun	Local distending pain
Shousanli (LI-10, on the affected side)	No. 30 filiform needle, 1.5 cun in length	Insert perpendicularly between the radius and the ulna to a depth of 0.5-0.8 cun	Local distending pain and/or pain radiating towards the thumb
Baxie (EX-UE-9, in the interspace between the second and third metacarpal, on the affected side)	No. 30 filiform needle, 2 cun in length	Insert parallel to the surface of the skin towards the wrist for about 1.8 cun	Local distending pain

Method
- The patient adopts a sitting position.
- The acupoints are needled with the needles being retained for 40 minutes; during this period, one session of needle manipulation takes place.

- Acupuncture is performed once a day for ten consecutive days (one course of treatment).
- Recommence the treatment after an interval of five days, if necessary.

Clinical notes

Clinically, apart from acupuncture, there is no specific effective treatment for this condition. During acupuncture, the patient should be advised not to be afraid of the pen, and writing should be temporarily suspended. After one course of treatment, the patient should be allowed to write a little; during the second course, the patient should write more and more until the condition is cured.

Chapter 4

Lower limb conditions

44 ISCHIAL BURSITIS

This condition is an aseptic inflammation of the ischial bursa, resulting from excessive pressure and friction, which gradually leads to a thickening or fibrosis of the synovial wall. It often occurs among people who sit for prolonged periods, and especially affects the middle-aged, the elderly, and weak people. It produces pain, and in a few cases injury to the buttocks results in regional swelling.

Clinical manifestations
- local swelling, tenderness, pain when sitting and raising the leg to climb stairs
- oval swollen mass with a defined margin in the deep layer of the ischial tuberosity, aggravated by movement and alleviated by rest
- in severe cases, pain extends along the distribution of the sciatic nerve

TREATMENT
Acupoints and techniques

Combination of points	Needles used	Insertion technique	Needling sensation
Tender area (on the affected side): A very obvious tender area is located in the region of the ischial tuberosity	Two no. 28 filiform needles, 3 cun in length	Insert to a depth of 2.5 cun at the sides of the tender area into the swollen mass in the ischial tuberosity	Regional distending pain or pain radiating to the lower limb
Zhibian (BL-54, on the affected side)	No. 30 filiform needle, 3 cun in length	Insert perpendicularly to a depth of 2.5 cun	Regional distending pain
Weizhong (BL-40, on the affected side)	No. 30 filiform needle, 2 cun in length	Insert perpendicularly to a depth of 1.0-1.2 cun	Regional distending pain

Method
- The patient lies in a prone position.
- The acupoints are needled with the needles being retained for 40 minutes; during this period, one session of needle manipulation takes place.

- After the needles are withdrawn, cupping therapy is performed for one minute.
- Acupuncture should be performed once a day; one course of treatment consists of ten sessions.
- An interval of five days is required between two courses of treatment.

Clinical notes

Acupuncture is reasonably effective in treating this condition. If there is a large effusion and mobile mass at the ischial tuberosity, corticosteroid injection should be considered in conjunction with acupuncture therapy. For patients with less effusion, ten or more acupuncture treatments may be required. After recovery or during treatment, patients should be advised to exercise the legs gently, and to avoid violent movement and sitting for long periods. Sitting on a soft cushion or a round air cushion is recommended. This condition has a tendency to relapse. When relapse occurs, treatment should be prompt. Acupuncture is generally a useful therapy in treating this disease.

45 PIRIFORMIS MUSCLE SYNDROME

This syndrome results from injury or overstrain of the piriformis muscle and pelvic inflammatory disease affecting the muscle, leading to entrapment of the sciatic nerve in the greater sciatic notch. Clinically, it is commonly encountered with sciatica.

Clinical manifestations
- pain occurs along the distribution of the sciatic nerve after exercise
- sensation of shortness of the affected limb, walking with a slight limp, painful and heavy sensation in the buttock, radiating pain over the regions behind the affected thigh and lateral to the shin, and hypoaesthesia of the skin
- in severe cases, there is obvious lameness of the affected limb
- gluteal pain radiates to the lower abdomen, the back of the thigh and the lateral side of the calf, accompanied by discomfort in the pudendum or sharp pain of the scrotum and testis
- pain occurs when the lower limbs are straightened and becomes sharp when the affected limb is in external rotation and flexion, or during coughing and sneezing; pain is alleviated after rest
- if the problem is prolonged, some patients may develop atrophy of the lateral muscles of the calf
- alleviation of pain during internal rotation of the affected limb and after movement

TREATMENT
Acupoints and techniques

Combination of points	Needles used	Insertion technique	Needling sensation
Huantiao (GB-30, on the affected side)	No. 30 filiform needle, 3.5 cun in length	Insert to a depth of 2.5-3.0 cun towards the piriformis muscle	Regional distending pain or pain radiating to the perineum or the lower limb and sole

Chengfu (BL-36, on the affected side)	No. 30 filiform needle, 2.5 cun in length	Insert perpendicularly to a depth of 2.0 cun	Regional distending pain
Yinmen (BL-37, on the affected side)	No. 30 filiform needle, 2.5 cun in length	Insert perpendicularly to a depth of 2.0 cun	Regional distending pain
Weizhong (BL-40, on the affected side)	No. 30 filiform needle, 2 cun in length	Insert perpendicularly to a depth of 1.0-1.2 cun	Regional distending pain

Method
- The patient lies in a prone position.
- The acupoints are needled with the needles being retained for 40 minutes; during this period, one session of needle manipulation takes place.
- After the needles are withdrawn, cupping therapy is performed for one minute.
- Acupuncture should be performed once a day; one course of treatment consists of ten sessions.
- An interval of five days is required between two courses of treatment.

Clinical notes
Acupuncture therapy is relatively effective in the treatment of the syndrome when caused by simple injury to the piriformis muscle. If it is accompanied by pelvic inflammatory disease, anti-inflammation treatment should be considered to achieve a better result. The pain caused by problems on the surface of the area inferior to the greater sciatic foramen should be distinguished from sciatica. Accurate diagnosis and precise selection of acupoints are essential to achieve a successful result.

46 TROCHANTERIC BURSITIS

This condition is generally caused by chronic injury and often occurs among weak and thin people as a result of prolonged lying on the side, resulting in friction and pressure between the gluteal aponeurosis and the greater trochanter of the femur. This produces aseptic inflammation. If the condition persists, organization of the effusion may occur.

Clinical manifestations
- pain and tenderness along the femur
- if the effusion increases, a painful nodular mass with a definite margin can be found at the greater trochanter
- pain occurs when the thigh is in flexion and internally rotated and is alleviated when it is in abduction and externally rotated

TREATMENT
Acupoints and techniques

Combination of points	Needles used	Insertion technique	Needling sensation
Regional tender area (on the affected side): Evident tenderness at the location of the bursa	No. 28 filiform needle, 2 cun in length	Insert to a depth of 1.5 cun in the direction of the neck of the femur	Regional distending pain
Huantiao (GB-30, on the affected side)	No. 30 filiform needle, 3.5 cun in length	Insert to a depth of 2.5-3.0 cun in the direction of the greater sciatic foramen	Regional distending pain or distending pain radiating to the sole
Chengfu (BL-36, on the affected side)	No. 30 filiform needle, 2.5 cun in length	Insert perpendicularly to a depth of 2.0 cun	Regional distending pain
Weizhong (BL-40, on the affected side)	No. 30 filiform needle, 2 cun in length	Insert perpendicularly to a depth of 1.0-1.2 cun	Regional distending pain

Method
- The patient lies in a prone position.
- The acupoints are needled with the needles being retained for 40 minutes; during this period, one session of needle manipulation takes place.
- After the needles are withdrawn, cupping therapy is performed for one minute.
- Acupuncture should be performed once a day; one course of treatment consists of ten sessions.
- An interval of five days is required between two courses of treatment.

Clinical notes
If there is significant effusion and obvious local mass, the fluid should be aspirated and a corticosteroid injection may be administered. The curative effect is satisfactory. At a more advanced stage of bursitis, characterized by the resolution of inflammation and continuation of local pain, acupuncture therapy should be used as described above. If there is a small amount of effusion, acupuncture alone is enough to deal with the bursitis.

47 SEQUELAE OF FRACTURE OF THE FEMORAL NECK

These symptoms are commonly encountered among elderly people after healing of a fracture of the femoral neck. Where this type of fracture occurs among young people, it is usually caused by serious injury, such as a vehicular accident or falling from a height.

A number of factors are associated with the sequelae of the fracture, including abnormal union of the fracture, bone necrosis, deformity, and errors of internal fixation of the fracture, laceration of the joint capsule, haemarthrosis within the hip joint capsule, or adhesion and contraction due to injury of the tissues around the joint capsule after surgery.

Clinical manifestations
- often seen among elderly patients with an obvious fracture or following surgery for fracture
- pain usually appears in the buttock and radiates to the leg
- pain is aggravated when the patient moves or turns over whilst asleep
- the patient usually walks slowly with a walking aid
- patients with abnormal union and bone necrosis usually feel that the affected limb is short; the pain becomes sharp on weight-bearing
- in severe cases, the pain may radiate to the lower limb, particularly to the territory of the sciatic nerve or the anterior cutaneous nerve of the thigh

Examination
- obvious tender area in the upper part of the femur
- obvious muscular atrophy in the buttock in persistent cases; the pain is aggravated when flexing or externally rotating the thigh and on weight-bearing
- in severe cases, radiating pain occurs in the lower limb when the tender area in the buttock is pressed
- X-ray examination shows an old fracture of the femoral neck or necrosis, deformity or abnormal union of the femoral head

TREATMENT
Acupoints and techniques

Combination of points	Needles used	Insertion technique	Needling sensation
Tender area (on the affected side): Two obvious tender areas can be located in the region between the greater trochanter and the hip joint	Two no. 28 filiform needles, 2 cun in length	Insert both needles to a depth of 1.5 cun in the tender areas towards the hip joint	Regional distending pain
Yinmen (BL-37, on the affected side)	No. 30 filiform needle, 2.5 cun in length	Insert perpendicularly to a depth of 2.0 cun	Regional distending pain
Weizhong (BL-40, on the affected side)	No. 30 filiform needle, 2 cun in length	Insert perpendicularly to a depth of 1.0-1.2 cun	Regional distending pain

Method
- The patient lies in a prone position.
- The acupoints are needled using electro-acupuncture, with the needles being retained for 40 minutes.
- After the needles are withdrawn, cupping therapy is performed for one minute.
- Acupuncture should be performed once a day; one course of treatment consists of ten sessions.
- An interval of five days is required between two courses of treatment.

Clinical notes
Electro-acupuncture is fairly effective in stopping pain and relieving local adhesions, but the treatment may take a long time. In this instance, the curative effect is often satisfactory. After the pain has been alleviated, patients should be advised to exercise their legs (starting with slow movement of the legs and progressing to slow walking and leisurely jogging) to promote rehabilitation. Exercise should not be too strenuous in order to avoid relapse.

48 INJURY TO THE VASTUS MEDIALIS MUSCLE

Injury produces sprain or tearing of the muscle, local blood stasis (according to TCM diagnosis) and oedema. It is often caused by an indirect force, such as gymnastics, doing the splits, running, and participating in high jumping and long jumping. In other cases, vehicular accidents or falling from a height may cause direct injury to the muscle and lead to blood stasis, oedema and pain in the affected area. If the above conditions persist, or there are climatic changes, distending discomfort over the affected region usually results.

Clinical manifestations
- pain and swelling over the origin of the muscle are the main symptoms in most patients with acute injury
- tumescent and distending pain can be found in the upper or lower third of the internal aspect of the thigh, in most cases resulting from direct external injury
- sharp pain can be felt in flexion of the knee and in external rotation, adduction and abduction of the thigh
- where the condition has persisted, obvious tenderness and a line of nodules are palpable over the upper or lower third of the internal aspect of the thigh

TREATMENT
Acupoints and techniques

Combination of points	Needles used	Insertion technique	Needling sensation
Tender area on the upper thigh (on the affected side): The most obvious swelling or tenderness is located on the upper third of the internal aspect of the thigh	Three no. 30 filiform needles, 2 cun in length	Insert perpendicularly to a depth of 1.5 cun into the tender area, avoiding obvious veins	Regional distending pain

Tender area on the lower thigh (on the affected side): Three obvious tender areas may be found on the lower third of the internal aspect of the thigh	Three no. 30 filiform needles, 2 cun in length	Insert perpendicularly to a depth of 1.3-1.5 cun, avoiding obvious veins	Regional distending pain
Xuehai (SP-10, on the affected side)	No. 30 filiform needle, 2 cun in length	Insert perpendicularly to a depth of 1.0-1.5 cun	Regional distending pain

Method

- The patient lies in a supine position.
- The acupoints are needled with the needles being retained for 40 minutes; during this period, one session of needle manipulation takes place.
- After the needles are withdrawn, cupping therapy is performed for one minute.
- Acupuncture should be performed once a day; one course of treatment consists of six sessions.
- An interval of three days is required between two courses of treatment.

Clinical notes

Acupuncture therapy has proved quite effective in treating injury to the vastus medialis muscle at an early stage. If there is local haematoma, needling therapy should not be undertaken until the haematoma resorbs. During the course of treatment, the patient should be advised to avoid excessive movement and to rest the affected limb on a comfortable surface. After the curative effect is felt, the patient is advised to do some gentle exercises, such as moving the legs up and down or walking, to promote rehabilitation.

49 SPRAIN OF THE QUADRICEPS FEMORIS

This condition is usually caused by injury to the quadriceps femoris while playing football or jumping or from injury to the thigh, resulting from a sudden contraction of the muscles and sprain at their origins.

Clinical manifestations
- at the early stage, pain or tenderness can be felt in the anterior inferior iliac spine and on the upper third of the anterior femur
- pain occurs on movement of the hip joint and extension of the knee three to five days after the injury is sustained. The pain is located in the distribution of the quadriceps femoris and at a later stage radiates throughout the quadriceps and to the knee and lower leg

Examination
- obvious tender area on the anterior inferior iliac spine, the superior part of the acetabulum, or the anterior femur
- aggravation of pain on extension of the thigh and knee

TREATMENT
Acupoints and techniques

Combination of points	Needles used	Insertion technique	Needling sensation
Qiaqianxiaji (inferior anterior iliac spine, on the affected side): Located 1 cun below the median point (Chongmen SP-12) of the inguinal ligament (see diagram, page 167)	No. 30 filiform needle, 2 cun in length	Insert to a depth of 1.5 cun towards the iliac bone	Regional distending pain
Biguan (ST-31, on the affected side)	No. 30 filiform needle, 2 cun in length	Insert obliquely (at an angle of 45°) to a depth of 1.5 cun into the internal lateral aspect of the thigh	Regional distending pain

Xuehai (SP-10, on the affected side)	No. 30 filiform needle, 2 cun in length	Insert perpendicularly to a depth of 1.0-1.5 cun	Regional distending pain
Xiguanjie (on the affected side): Located two finger-widths directly above the median point of the upper margin of the patella (see diagram, page 167)	No. 30 filiform needle, 3 cun in length	Insert to a depth of 2.5 cun towards the internal lateral aspect of the thigh at an angle of 25° between the needle and the skin	Regional distending pain

Method

- The patient lies in a supine position.
- The acupoints are needled with the needles being retained for 40 minutes; during this period, one session of needle manipulation takes place.
- After the needles are withdrawn, cupping therapy is performed for one minute.
- Acupuncture should be performed once a day; one course of treatment consists of ten sessions.
- An interval of five days is required between two courses of treatment.

Clinical notes

Injury to the quadriceps femoris can be treated effectively by needling therapy. If the patient is at an advanced stage of a persistent condition, needling therapy should be used in combination with electro-acupuncture. The curative effect is satisfactory in these cases as well.

50 NEURITIS OF THE LATERAL CUTANEOUS NERVE OF THE THIGH (MERALGIA PARAESTHETICA)

This condition, which is also known as Bernhardt's disease, Bernhardt-Roth syndrome or Roth-Bernhardt disease, is precipitated by compression or injury of the nerve at sites along its course.

Aetiologically, two types are recognized: primary and secondary. The causes of the former are not clear in most cases. The latter are secondary to systemic and, more especially, local diseases or conditions, such as injuries or entrapment of the nerve at the inguinal ligament. Other causes include nerve compression due to increased soft tissue bulk during pregnancy and wearing clothing that is too tight.

Clinical manifestations
- prevalent in middle-aged and obese males, or women during pregnancy and after childbirth
- usually unilateral
- symptoms include numbness, stabbing pain, burning sensation, formication, and burning pain in the lower two-thirds of the anterior lateral side of the thigh
- symptoms are aggravated after standing up or walking for a long time; symptoms may also be exacerbated in obese patients when they sit down
- the disease can be self-limiting and is likely to recur

Examination
- hypoaesthesia or hyperaesthesia to painful stimuli, touch or temperature can be found on the lateral side of the thigh, sometimes with tender points
- no muscular atrophy, and tendon reflexes are normal

TREATMENT
Acupoints and techniques
Five-needle acupuncture at tenderness acupoints
The location of the tender points on the lateral aspect of the lower thigh cannot be specified exactly. Since most patients cannot indicate the tender points accurately, the location refers to an area of discomfort, numbness or pain. Having identified the overall area indicated by the patient, select five points in a circumference 1 cm larger than this area. One point will be in the centre of the area, the others being situated above, below and to the right and left of the area (see diagram I, page 168).

Five no. 30 filiform needles, 2 cun in length, are inserted sequentially in the upper, inner, lower, outer and central points. The first four needles are all directed towards the centre and the central needle is inserted perpendicularly to the surface of the skin.

A distending pain is felt, along with a sensation of tightening up towards the central point.

Method
- The patient lies in a supine position.
- The acupoints are needled with the needles being retained for 40 minutes; during this period, one session of needle manipulation takes place.
- Cupping therapy is performed for one minute immediately after the needles are removed.
- Acupuncture is performed once a day for ten consecutive days (one course of treatment).
- Recommence the treatment after an interval of five days, if necessary.

Clinical notes
Acupuncture treatment is very effective for this condition, which can generally be cured after eight to ten sessions. However, in some cases, the disease can recur when patients catch cold or are of a weak constitution or experience excessive uterine bleeding during menstruation. The therapy is also satisfactory after recurrence. After recovery, the patient should be advised to avoid known precipitating factors and increase physical exercise to avoid recurrence.

51 LESION OF THE INFRAPATELLAR FAT PAD

This is one of the most commonly-encountered knee problems, mainly resulting from violent or prolonged movement of the knee.

It frequently occurs among obese middle-aged or elderly women, and is
usually caused by repeated sprain, jarring and prolonged loading of the knee,
which gradually lead to oedema and organization of the tissues as well as
degenerative changes and gradual thickening of the tissues, together with swelling and pain.

Clinical manifestations
- distending pain when standing, squatting or hyperextending the knee
- weakness of the knee when walking, tumescent pain and distension of the
  infrapatellar ligament and knee
- obvious tenderness
- aversion to cold and draughts in some patients

Examination
- obvious tenderness below the lower pole of the patella
- knee hyperextension test is positive: the patient lies flat and extends the patellar joint. The doctor grasps the ankle of the affected limb while pressing the
  knee with the other hand to hyperextend it. If pain occurs at the infrapatellar
  fat pad area, the test is positive
- positive relaxed patellar tendon test: the patient lies flat and fully extends the
  knee. The doctor puts the thumb of one hand on the knee, while placing the
  palm of the other hand on the dorsum of the patient's big toe. The patient
  relaxes the quadriceps and the doctor gradually presses the big toe. Pain may
  be felt when pressure is applied. The patient is then asked to flex the quadriceps and the doctor reapplies the pressure. If the pain is alleviated, this
  means the relaxed patellar tendon test is positive

TREATMENT
Acupoints and techniques

Combination of points	Needles used	Insertion technique	Needling sensation
Neixiyan (EX-LE-4) and Dubi (ST-35, on the affected side)	Two no. 28 filiform needles, 1.5 cun in length	Insert to a depth of 0.5-1.0 cun in the centre of the area	Regional distending pain and distending sensation over ST-35 radiating to the dorsum of the foot
Heding (EX-LE-2, on the affected side)	No. 30 filiform needle, 2 cun in length	Insert obliquely upwards (at an angle of 45°) to a depth of 0.8-1.2 cun	Regional distending pain or pain radiating to the upper region of the femur
Zusanli (ST-36, on the affected side)	No. 30 filiform needle, 2.5 cun in length	Insert perpendicularly to a depth of 1.8 cun	Regional distending pain or pain radiating to the dorsum of the foot

Method
- The patient adopts a sitting position.
- The acupoints are needled with the needles being retained for 40 minutes; during this period, one session of needle manipulation takes place.
- After the needles are withdrawn, cupping therapy is performed for one minute.
- Acupuncture should be performed once a day; one course of treatment consists of ten sessions.
- An interval of five days is required between two courses of treatment.

Clinical notes
Acupuncture therapy has proven effective in treating lesions of the infrapatellar fat pad, especially at the acute stage. A longer course of treatment is required for patients who have suffered from the condition for a long period, but the curative effect is also satisfactory. During treatment, the patient should avoid violent movement and strain of the knee, for example by pulling a load or squatting.

52 PREPATELLAR BURSITIS (HOUSEMAID'S KNEE)

This condition usually results from acute or chronic injury or local infection. Acute injury produces local swelling and an effusion in the bursa; chronic injury is associated with prolonged friction, pressure or stimulation and slight trauma of the patella. If the patient has a weak constitution, abnormal climatic changes and changes in air pressure may result in an increase in effusion in a previously-damaged bursa. Suppurative bursitis is due to spread of skin infection or involvement of the bursa by open traumatic infection.

Clinical manifestations
- obvious traumatic history in acute cases, resulting in local swelling and obvious tenderness
- at an advanced stage, gradual disappearance of swelling in surrounding tissues, but obvious persistence of swelling and tenderness over the prepatellar bursa
- in chronic cases, there may be a gradual onset with no obvious history of trauma
- pain restricted to the prepatellar bursa
- progressive effusion, and tumescent and distending pain at the advanced stage
- infective bursitis is characterized by the appearance of infection followed by inflammatory swelling and distension of the bursa

Examination
- mobile swelling of the prepatellar bursa
- obvious tenderness and no change in swelling over the knee when lifting the legs

TREATMENT
Acupoints and techniques

Combination of points	Needles used	Insertion technique	Needling sensation
Neixiyan (EX-LE-4) and Dubi (ST-35, on the affected side)	Two no. 28 filiform needles, 1.5 cun in length	Insert to a depth of 0.5-1.0 cun in the centre of the area	Regional distending pain and distending sensation over ST-35 radiating to the dorsum of the foot
Heding (EX-LE-2, on the affected side)	No. 30 filiform needle, 1.5 cun in length	Insert perpendicularly to a depth of 0.5-1.0 cun	Regional distending pain
Zusanli (ST-36, on the affected side)	No. 30 filiform needle, 2.5 cun in length	Insert perpendicularly to a depth of 1.8 cun	Regional distending pain or pain radiating to the dorsum of the foot

Method
- The patient adopts a sitting position.
- The acupoints are needled, with the needles being retained for 40 minutes; during this period, one session of needle manipulation is carried out.
- After the needles are withdrawn, cupping therapy is performed for one minute.
- Acupuncture should be performed once a day; one course of treatment consists of ten sessions.
- An interval of five days is required between two courses of treatment.

Clinical notes
Acupuncture therapy is applicable and effective where there is no effusion and only local pain or pain after movement. It cannot be used when there is an effusion. At this stage, the effusion must be aspirated first. This therapy has proven effective. Where there is infection, antibiotic therapy should be used first.

53 POPLITEAL CYST (BAKER'S CYST)

Popliteal cyst is a synovial sac in continuity with the knee joint. It develops in patients with chronic knee arthritis and causes progressive distension in the popliteal fossa. Occasionally the cyst leaks into the calf causing pain and swelling which may be confused with deep venous thrombosis. Popliteal cyst must be distinguished from an aneurysm of the popliteal artery: the latter is pulsatile.

Clinical manifestations
- history of chronic arthritis of the knee
- the cyst enlarges slowly
- at the initial stage, no symptoms or just slight discomfort of the knee, which is often overlooked
- when there is obvious swelling, symptoms include dull pain, discomfort, weakness of the lower limb, restriction of knee flexion, and weakness of the knee after prolonged walking or on climbing stairs
- if the weather and air pressure change, the patient may feel increased swelling
- if the cyst enlarges, it may press on the vein and cause distal varicosity; the patient may then feel distension of the lower leg when standing

Examination
- obvious cystic swelling in the popliteal fossa
- in some patients at an early stage, the cyst can be compressed without producing tenderness
- when the knee extends, the cyst becomes more prominent and firmer; when the knee flexes, it becomes less prominent and softer

TREATMENT
Acupoints and techniques

Combination of points	Needles used	Insertion technique	Needling sensation
Tender area: Locate the highest point of the cyst in the popliteal fossa on the affected side, followed by the four margins of the cyst (see diagram II, page 168)	Five no. 28 filiform needles, 2 cun in length	Under strict sterile conditions, one needle is inserted to a depth of 1.0 cun into the centre of the cyst and the other four needles are inserted to a depth of 1.5 cun at the median points of the four cyst margins	Regional distending pain

Method
- The patient lies in a prone position.
- The acupoints are needled with the needles being retained for 40 minutes; during this period, one session of needle manipulation takes place.
- After the needles are withdrawn, cupping therapy is performed for one minute.
- Acupuncture should be performed once every other day; one course of treatment consists of six sessions.
- Treatment should be stopped if it is ineffective.

Clinical notes
This therapy is effective in treating popliteal fossa cyst at an early stage or a cyst without adhesions and inflammation. Some patients will suffer relapse, which can be treated in the same way. Where there is obvious inflammation of the cyst wall, the patient should be advised to consult Western medicine specialists first. When the inflammation has subsided, needling therapy can be applied. Joint aspiration may be considered in cases of persistent popliteal cyst.

54 TRAUMATIC SYNOVITIS OF THE KNEE

The main symptom of this condition, which can be acute or chronic traumatic inflammation, is haemarthrosis of the knee joint. Chronic traumatic synovitis occurs more frequently among women, especially obese women.

The condition results from acute trauma, chronic arthritis, rheumatic arthritis, rheumatoid arthritis, gout, suppurative arthritis, tuberculous arthritis, or pigmented villonodular synovitis. The synovial membrane secretes increased quantities of fluid and there may be intra-articular bleeding, resulting in swelling of the joint, and restricted flexion and extension of the joint. In severe cases, adhesions may cause dysfunction of the joint.

Clinical manifestations

Acute injury:
- characterized by the development of haematoma and painful swelling of the knee joint either immediately or within one to two hours
- full knee flexion and extension is impaired
- if there is haemarthrosis, the colour of the blood alters with time as the pigment is resorbed

Chronic injury:
- usually caused by inappropriate treatment of acute bursitis
- often seen among elderly, obese people
- at an early stage, the patient usually has an aversion to cold and wind, and experiences discomfort, heaviness, fluctuant swelling and pain of the knee joint
- if the condition persists, the pain is exacerbated by squatting
- in patients with osteophyte formation, there may be valgus or varus deformity of the knee
- in some chronic cases affecting debilitated patients (for example, where suffering from fever, diarrhoea or a cold), the synovial secretion may increase, causing a tense effusion

TREATMENT
Acupoints and techniques

Combination of points	Needles used	Insertion technique	Needling sensation
Neixiyan (EX-LE-4) and Dubi (ST-35, on the affected side)	Two no. 28 filiform needles, 1.5 cun in length	Insert to a depth of 0.5-1.0 cun in the centre of the area	Regional distending pain and distending sensation over ST-35 radiating to the dorsum of the foot
Xuehai (SP-10, on the affected side)	No. 30 filiform needle, 2 cun in length	Insert perpendicularly to a depth of 1.0-1.5 cun	Regional distending pain
Xiguanjie (on the affected side): Located two finger-widths directly above the median point of the upper margin of the patella (see diagram, page 167)	No. 30 filiform needle, 2 cun in length	Insert obliquely upwards (at an angle of 45°) to a depth of 1.5 cun	Local distending pain or pain radiating to the knee joint
Zusanli (ST-36, on the affected side)	No. 30 filiform needle, 2.5 cun in length	Insert perpendicularly to a depth of 1.8 cun	Regional distending pain or pain radiating to the dorsum of the foot

Method
- The patient adopts a sitting position.
- The acupoints are needled with the needles being retained for 40 minutes; during this period, one session of needle manipulation takes place.
- After the needles are withdrawn, cupping therapy is performed for one minute.
- Acupuncture should be performed once a day; one course of treatment consists of ten sessions.
- An interval of five days is required between two courses of treatment.

Clinical notes

Acupuncture therapy can be performed on patients with a small effusion or where there is no suppurative inflammation. Several courses of treatment are required to treat chronic traumatic synovitis. If there is a haemarthrosis, the effusion should be aspirated and intra-articular steroid may be injected into the knee. Only when the effusion has been satisfactorily treated can needling therapy be used.

Suppurative arthritis is a serious condition requiring antibiotic treatment under specialist care. Needling therapy can only be used after eradication of the infection to eliminate adhesions and pain in the quadriceps muscle and the joint capsule.

Exercise is essential at a later stage to treat this condition effectively. This generally begins after the relief of pain and mainly concentrates on quadriceps exercises to prevent atrophy, and flexion and extension exercises for the knee to prevent loss of joint function.

55 INJURY TO THE TIBIAL COLLATERAL LIGAMENT OF THE KNEE

This condition is commonly seen and is encountered in labourers and athletes. The main symptom is pain over the medial aspect of the knee and the adjacent areas of the lower femur and upper tibia.

The main cause of this injury is forced abduction of the lower leg accompanied by rotation of the knee during sporting activities and vehicular accidents. In mild cases, the ligament is stretched or may be partially torn. Serious injury is rare but may result in injury to the meniscus and cruciate ligaments.

A few patients with an injury of this ligament may feel only slight local pain at the medial condylar attachment. Calcification and heterotopic ossification (myositis ossificans) may develop in the surrounding tissues.

Clinical manifestations
- obvious history of forced abduction injury of the lower leg with rotation of the knee
- in mild cases, pain is located on the medial aspect of the knee and a tender area can be found during sports and under pressure; pain is relieved after rest
- in severe cases, there is painful local swelling
- where the ligament is torn, there may be subcutaneous haematoma and unbearable pain during sports activities, getting out of bed, and going up and down stairs, together with instability of the joint
- at the later stage, local swelling and bruising disappear, but tenderness is obvious and pain becomes sharp when going up and down stairs
- X-ray examination: Plain films may show avulsion of a small fragment of bone. Films taken with abduction of the knee (under anaesthesia if necessary) may demonstrate opening of the joint space. Heterotopic calcification or bone formation (myositis ossificans) may be seen
- MRI scan or arthroscopy may be necessary to establish whether the meniscus or cruciate ligaments have been damaged

TREATMENT
Acupoints and techniques

Combination of points	Needles used	Insertion technique	Needling sensation
Tender area: Obvious tenderness can be found in the area of the tibial collateral ligament on the affected side	Three no. 28 filiform needles, 2 cun in length	With the tender area as the centre, insert the needles in a fan shape to a depth of 1.5 cun towards the quadriceps femoris	Regional distending pain
Xuehai (SP-10, on the affected side)	No. 30 filiform needle, 2 cun in length	Insert perpendicularly to a depth of 1.0-1.5 cun	Regional distending pain
Yinlingquan (SP-9, on the affected side)	No. 28 filiform needle, 2 cun in length	Insert perpendicularly to the tibia to a depth of 1.2-1.5 cun	Regional distending pain

Method
- The patient adopts a sitting position.
- The acupoints are needled, with the needles being retained for 40 minutes; during this period, one session of needle manipulation is carried out.
- After the needles are withdrawn, cupping therapy is performed for one minute.
- Acupuncture should be performed once a day; one course of treatment consists of six sessions.
- If there is no effect, corticosteroid injection can be considered.

Clinical notes
Acupuncture therapy is effective in the treatment of mild injury or injury at an early stage. The best effect is generally achieved when treatment is given within one week of the injury. The result is not satisfactory two weeks or more after the injury. Corticosteroid injection can be used if acupuncture treatment does not give satisfactory results. Acupuncture cannot be undertaken on patients with ruptured ligaments and severe meniscal injury or cruciate damage; these situations require orthopaedic assessment and appropriate management. If an operation is required, needling therapy is effective in relieving post-operative pain.

56 INJURY TO THE FIBULAR COLLATERAL LIGAMENT OF THE KNEE

This injury is much less common than injury to the tibial collateral ligament. The main symptom is swelling and pain of the fibular collateral ligament.

The principal cause of this injury is sudden forced adduction of the lower leg accompanied by internal rotation of the lower leg during sporting activities and vehicular accidents, particularly when the knee is in partial flexion. In serious cases, there may be partial or complete rupture of the fibular collateral ligament, damage to the lateral joint capsule, the arcuate popliteal ligament, the cruciate ligaments, the biceps femoris muscle, the tendon of the popliteus muscle, and the common peroneal nerve.

Clinical manifestations
- local swelling and pain in mild cases
- pain when climbing stairs, alleviation after rest
- in severe cases, local haematoma and swelling anterior to the fibula; if the joint capsule is stretched, a haemarthrosis may develop
- partial or complete tearing of the ligament, or internal joint derangement, causing instability of the knee joint
- injury to the common peroneal nerve results in foot-drop and sensory disturbance over the fibula and the medial part of the dorsum of the foot
- X-ray examination: Plain films may show avulsion of a small fragment of bone. Films taken with adduction of the knee (under anaesthesia if necessary) may demonstrate opening of the joint space
- MRI scan or arthroscopy may be necessary to establish whether the meniscus or cruciate ligaments have been damaged

TREATMENT
Acupoints and techniques

Combination of points	Needles used	Insertion technique	Needling sensation
Tender area (on the affected side): Obvious tenderness located in the region of the fibular collateral ligament	No. 28 filiform needle, 2.5 cun in length	Insert obliquely to a depth of 1.8 cun along the collateral ligament towards the popliteal fossa	Regional distending pain
Yanglingquan (GB-34, on the affected side)	No. 30 filiform needle, 2 cun in length	Insert perpendicularly, then move the needle parallel to the skin for 1.2-1.5 cun along the tibiofibular articulation	Regional distending pain or pain radiating to the dorsum of the foot
Tiaokou (ST-38, on the affected side)	No. 30 filiform needle, 2.5 cun in length	Insert perpendicularly to a depth of 1.8 cun	Regional distending pain or pain radiating to the dorsum of the foot
Xiangu (ST-43, on the affected side)	No. 30 filiform needle, 1.5 cun in length	Insert slightly perpendicularly (at an angle of 75°) to a depth of 1.0 cun	Regional distending pain

Method
- The patient adopts a sitting position.
- The acupoints are needled using electro-acupuncture, with the needles being retained for 40 minutes; during this period, one session of needle manipulation is carried out.
- After the needles are withdrawn, cupping therapy is performed for one minute.
- Acupuncture should be performed once a day; one course of treatment consists of ten sessions.
- An interval of five days is required between two courses of treatment.

Clinical notes
Most cases of this injury are serious and require management by an orthopaedic surgeon. Where there is injury to the cruciate ligament or haemarthrosis, needling therapy should be suspended until absorption of the haemarthrosis. Acupuncture therapy is effective in treating the pain caused by the injury. If the case is a mild sprain of the fibular collateral ligament accompanied by local pain, the therapeutic method described above is very effective. However, if the effect is not satisfactory, corticosteroid injection should be considered.

57 INJURY TO THE SEMILUNAR CARTILAGE OF THE KNEE JOINT

This injury is common. The main symptoms are due to laceration of the lateral or medial meniscus, with damage to the joint capsule and the surrounding tissues.

The injury results from rotation of the lower leg when weight-bearing. It often appears among footballers, basketball players, high-jumpers and discus throwers. It may also occur among people who squat at work and are therefore liable to chronic knee strain.

Clinical manifestations
- pain results from weight-bearing
- regional distending and tumescent pain and snapping pain

The injury can be classified as follows:

Physical exertion:
- pain mainly occurs during movement or going up and down stairs
- pain is at its worst when exertion is at its greatest

After the injury:
- swelling, and local distending and tumescent pain in the region of the meniscus

Mild injury:
- flexion and extension of the knee joint may not be affected
- a click may accompany flexion and extension of the knee

Serious injury:
- the joint may "lock" suddenly during sports or other activities; this is manifested by an inability to extend the knee fully and may be painful
- the injury is accompanied by an effusion with positive patellar tap sign
- MRI scan or arthroscopy may be required to assess meniscal damage

TREATMENT
Acupoints and techniques

Combination of points	Needles used	Insertion technique	Needling sensation
Neixiyan (EX-LE-4) and Dubi (ST-35, on the affected side)	Two no. 28 filiform needles, 1.5 cun in length	Insert to a depth of 0.5-1.0 cun in the centre of the area	Regional distending pain and distending sensation over ST-35 radiating to the dorsum of the foot

Xuehai (SP-10, on the affected side)	No. 30 filiform needle, 2 cun in length	Insert perpendicularly to a depth of 1.0-1.5 cun	Regional distending pain
Heding (EX-LE-2, on the affected side)	No. 30 filiform needle, 1.5 cun in length	Insert obliquely upwards (at an angle of 45°) to a depth of 0.5-1.0 cun towards Futu (ST-32)	Regional distending pain
Zusanli (ST-36, on the affected side)	No. 30 filiform needle, 2.5 cun in length	Insert perpendicularly to a depth of 1.8 cun	Regional distending pain or pain radiating to the dorsum of the foot

Method
- The patient adopts a sitting position.
- The acupoints are needled, with the needles being retained for 40 minutes; during this period, one session of needle manipulation is carried out.
- After the needles are withdrawn, cupping therapy is performed for one minute.
- Acupuncture should be performed once a day; one course of treatment consists of ten sessions.
- An interval of five days is required between two courses of treatment.

Clinical notes
Needling therapy is only effective at the initial stage in reducing swelling and relieving pain. It cannot be used when the injury is accompanied by effusion. An operation is sometimes required. Needling therapy can be used to reduce adhesions and alleviate pain during post-operative rehabilitation.

58 INJURY TO THE GASTROCNEMIUS MUSCLE

This injury may be caused by strong contraction of the gastrocnemius muscle in strenuous sports, such as running, jumping or playing tennis, or by chronic strain or dorsiflexion of the ankle joint. The injury can involve three distinct parts of the muscle: the origin of the gastrocnemius muscle, the belly of the gastrocnemius where it merges with the gastrocnemius tendon, and partial or complete rupture of the Achilles tendon (tendo calcaneus).

Clinical manifestations

Acute injury:
- history of recent trauma, local bruising and swelling with associated tenderness; pain aggravated in the tendon area during sports
- extensive subcutaneous ecchymosis, sensation of nodules on the bellies of the muscle with a hollow in the middle
- marked pain on weight-bearing
- in serious cases, inability to plantarflex the foot

Chronic injury:
- often occurs in the section of muscle adjacent to the femoral condyles or in the Achilles tendon
- no obvious swelling at the affected location
- injury to the Achilles tendon results in a visible and palpable gap 5 cm above the insertion of the tendon
- Simmond's test should be checked if there is a suspicion of tendon rupture: with the patient prone, the doctor squeezes the calf muscles. If the tendon is intact, the foot plantarflexes; if the tendon is ruptured, the foot does not move
- muscular atrophy in patients with prolonged injury

TREATMENT
Acupoints and techniques

Combination of points	Needles used	Insertion technique	Needling sensation
Tender area I (on the affected side): Obvious tenderness can be found at a location 1.5 cun below Weiyang (BL-39)	No. 28 filiform needle, 2.5 cun in length	Insert to a depth of 1.8 cun towards the tibia	Regional distending pain or pain radiating to the dorsum of the foot

Tender area II (on the affected side): Obvious tenderness can be found at a location 1 cun below Yingu (KI-10)	No. 30 filiform needle, 2.5 cun in length	Insert to a depth of 1.8 cun towards the fibula	Regional distending pain
Weizhong (BL-40, on the affected side)	No. 30 filiform needle, 2 cun in length	Insert perpendicularly to a depth of 1.0-1.5 cun	Regional distending pain
Chengjin (BL-56, on the affected side)	No. 30 filiform needle, 2 cun in length	Insert perpendicularly to a depth of 1.5 cun	Regional distending pain
Chengshan (BL-57, on the affected side)	No. 30 filiform needle, 2 cun in length	Insert perpendicularly to a depth of 1.5 cun	Regional distending pain

Method

- The patient lies in a prone position.
- The acupoints are needled, with the needles being retained for 40 minutes; during this period, one session of needle manipulation is carried out.
- After the needles are withdrawn, cupping therapy is performed for one minute.
- Acupuncture should be performed once a day; one course of treatment consists of six sessions.
- An interval of three days is required between two courses of treatment.

Clinical notes

Acupuncture is effective in treating injury to the gastrocnemius muscle, especially in treating injury to the origin of the muscle and the musculotendinous area. Where there are complications or in the case of simple lacerations, longer treatment is required, but the curative effect is also satisfactory. During or after treatment, certain regions of the leg remain sensitive to cold and liable to cramp. Patients should be advised to keep warm.

59 ANKLE JOINT LIGAMENT INJURY

This injury is caused by sudden inversion or eversion of the ankle joint, due for example to an unexpected force being exerted on the foot as a result of uneven ground underfoot or missing the step when going downstairs.

Inversion of the ankle mainly causes injury to the anterior talofibular and calcaneofibular ligaments, whereas eversion damages the deltoid ligament. Since the deltoid ligament is strong, it is unlikely to rupture.

Ankle joint ligament injury may result in rupture of the ligament or an avulsion fracture of the corresponding malleolus. There may be ecchymosis in the skin. Dislocation of the ankle joint may occur with severe damage to the ligaments.

Clinical manifestations
- obvious history of ankle joint injury
- the location of the pain and swelling depend on the type of injury; inversion injury results in damage to the lateral ankle whereas eversion injury results in damage to the medial ankle
- in mild cases, there is only distending pain below the malleolus; pain is exacerbated while weight-bearing
- in severe cases, there is ecchymosis, pain exacerbated by ankle movement, and swelling below the malleolus
- fracture dislocation of the ankle results in the rapid onset of swelling, and deformity may be marked

Examination
- obvious swelling and tenderness over the injured ligament
- X-ray may show an avulsion fracture of the malleolus; if there is concern about severe ligament damage, strain films should be obtained (under general anaesthesia if necessary) to establish whether talar tilt is present

TREATMENT
Acupoints and techniques

Combination of points	Needles used	Insertion technique	Needling sensation
Shenmai (BL-62, on the affected side)	No. 28 filiform needle, 0.5 cun in length	Insert perpendicularly to a depth of 0.3 cun	Regional distending pain

Kunlun (BL-60, on the affected side)	No. 30 filiform needle, 1.5 cun in length	Insert perpendicularly to a depth of 0.5-1.0 cun	Regional distending pain or pain radiating to the sole of the foot
Diwuhui (GB-42, on the affected side)	No. 30 filiform needle, 1.5 cun in length	Insert slightly obliquely perpendicularly upwards (at an angle of 75°) to a depth of 0.5-0.8 cun	Regional distending pain
Zhaohai (KI-6, on the affected side)	No. 30 filiform needle, 1 cun in length	Insert perpendicularly to a depth of 0.3-0.5 cun	Regional distending pain

Method
- The patient adopts a sitting position.
- The acupoints are needled, with the needles being retained for 40 minutes; during this period, one session of needle manipulation is carried out.
- After the needles are withdrawn, cupping therapy is performed for one minute.
- Acupuncture should be performed once a day; one course of treatment consists of six sessions.
- The treatment is continued until full recovery of the patient.

Clinical notes
Acupuncture is very effective in treating ankle ligament injury. The injury is usually cured after three to five sessions. During treatment, the patient is advised to avoid strenuous activity. The affected foot should be elevated above the level of the other parts of the body at rest. If the injury requires orthopaedic management, needling therapy should be used after this management is completed.

60 TARSAL TUNNEL SYNDROME

This relatively uncommon syndrome is caused by compression of the posterior tibial nerve within the tarsal tunnel.

The main causes are chronic dorsiflexion of the foot, repeated sprain of the ankle joint, increased venous pressure in the legs due to incompetent veins, cyst, eversion of the foot, and osteoma of the medial malleolus. These phenomena affect the tendons, nerves and vessels in the tarsal tunnel.

Clinical manifestations
- usually seen among youths and adults, especially male runners and jumpers, as well as people who stand for prolonged periods
- obesity may be a predisposing factor in women
- the disorder is slow at the onset; at the early stage, slight discomfort, alleviated after rest, is felt in the region of the medial malleolus after prolonged standing or during walking, running or jumping
- after prolonged nerve entrapment, patients may feel a numb or scorching painful sensation over the internal side of the heel, extending from the sole to the toes, especially at night
- in severe cases, there may be dry and shiny skin, and muscular atrophy in the sole

Examination
- mild swelling, local tenderness
- hard, fusiform swelling posterior to the medial malleolus
- sensory impairment in the sensory branches of the posterior tibial nerve supplying the foot and other main branches, such as the medial and lateral plantar nerves
- pain and numbness may also be aggravated by activities such as passive dorsiflexion and eversion of the foot or resisted plantar flexion
- electromyography may show fibrillation of the small plantar muscles
- nerve conduction studies may confirm the features of nerve entrapment within the tarsal tunnel

TREATMENT
Acupoints and techniques

Combination of points	Needles used	Insertion technique	Needling sensation
Zhaohai (KI-6, on the affected side)	No. 30 filiform needle, 1 cun in length	Insert perpendicularly to a depth of 0.3-0.5 cun	Regional distending pain
Taichong (LR-3, on the affected side)	No. 30 filiform needle, 1.5 cun in length	Insert obliquely upwards (at an angle of 45°) to a depth of 1.0 cun	Regional distending pain
Sanyinjiao (SP-6, on the affected side)	No. 30 filiform needle, 2 cun in length	Insert perpendicularly to a depth of 1.0-1.5 cun towards Xuanzhong (GB-39)	Regional distending pain
Rangu (KI-2, on the affected side)	No. 30 filiform needle, 1.5 cun in length	Insert perpendicularly to a depth of 1.0 cun	Regional distending pain

Method
- The patient adopts a sitting position.
- The acupoints are needled, with the needles being retained for 40 minutes; during this period, one session of needle manipulation is carried out.
- After the needles are withdrawn, cupping therapy is performed for one minute.
- Acupuncture should be performed once a day; one course of treatment consists of six sessions.
- An interval of three days is required between two courses of treatment.

Clinical notes
Acupuncture therapy is reasonably effective in treating tarsal tunnel syndrome. The syndrome is usually cured after three to five sessions. However, a longer course of treatment is required to treat patients who have been suffering from the syndrome for a prolonged period, where the syndrome is severe, or where the sole is numb. Patients should be advised to elevate the affected limb above the level of the rest of the body when they are resting or sleeping. Patients should rest as much as possible and avoid strenuous activity.

61 PLANTAR PAIN

Plantar pain is associated with compression of the phalangeal nerve.

It is mainly seen in cases with weakness of the foot muscles, ligamentous laxity, fallen transverse arch and chronic strain, or underdevelopment of the first tarsal bone and hallux valgus. Walking and standing generally cause pain in the distal end of one or more metatarsal bones.

Clinical manifestations
- pain in the tarsal bone is often felt when tired or after prolonged walking
- pain is generally felt in the head of the third and fourth tarsal bones, worse when weight-bearing; the pain is alleviated by redistributing weight on the foot
- pain appears burning or lancinating, and may radiate to the tip of the toes or even involve the leg in severe cases
- the dorsum of the foot may feel swollen

Examination
- obvious tenderness in the interosseous space with radiating pain or swelling
- X-ray indicates damage to the metatarsal tuberosity and the articular surface in some patients

TREATMENT
Acupoints and techniques

Combination of points	Needles used	Insertion technique	Needling sensation
Tender area (on the affected side): Obvious tenderness can be located in the intertarsal space between the third and fourth metatarsal bones or in other interosseous spaces	No. 30 filiform needles (the number used is based on the number of tender areas located), 1.5 cun in length	Insert to a depth of 0.5-1.0 cun in the sole	Distending pain over the dorsum and sole of the foot
Bafeng (EX-LE-10, on the affected side): See below	No. 30 filiform needles, 1 cun in length	Insert obliquely (at an angle of 45°) in the tender area to a depth of 0.3-0.5 cun	Regional distending pain

Note: Bafeng (EX-LE-10) is located on the interphalangeal spaces from the first to the fifth digits and at the junction of the red and white skin proximal to the interphalangeal webs. There are four acupoints on each side. The number of acupoints is determined by the number of tender areas chosen.

Method
- The patient adopts a sitting position.
- The acupoints are needled, with the needles being retained for 40 minutes; during this period, one session of needle manipulation is carried out.
- After the needles are withdrawn, cupping therapy is performed for one minute.
- Acupuncture should be performed once a day; one course of treatment consists of six sessions.
- An interval of three days is required between two courses of treatment.

Clinical notes
This acupuncture therapy is effective in treating tarsal pain. With accurate selection of the acupoints and proper technique, the pain can be cured in just four to five treatments. Patients should be advised to be careful when walking, and to avoid spraining the foot, injuring the sole or walking for a long time with a heavy load. To avoid relapse, patients should wear low-heeled shoes and correct their posture when placing their feet on the ground.

62 SEQUELAE OF ACHILLES TENDON RUPTURE

Rupture of the Achilles tendon is caused by violent injury to the heel and can be divided into complete and incomplete tears (see also section 58 on injury to the gastrocnemius muscle). Acupuncture therapy is best suited to post-operative sequelae or sequelae from treatments other than surgery.

Clinical manifestations
- post-operative scar contraction
- weakness and atrophy of the triceps surae muscle (the combined gastrocnemius and soleus muscles) and swelling of the Achilles tendon resulting from inappropriate exercise during rehabilitation
- pain in the heel when walking and distending pain in the heel in dorsiflexion or plantar flexion

Examination
- obvious surgical scars or depression over the affected part of a ruptured tendon treated conservatively
- obvious local swelling and tenderness, weakness of the triceps surae muscle in plantar flexion, or obvious atrophy of this muscle

TREATMENT
Acupoints and techniques

Combination of points	Needles used	Insertion technique	Needling sensation
Tender area (on the affected side): Two obvious tender areas can be located on the medial and lateral sides of the upper section of the Achilles tendon (in patients with surgical scars, the tenderness is located above and below the scars or on the medial and lateral sides of the scars)	Two no. 30 filiform needles, 1.5 cun in length	Insert perpendicularly to a depth of 1.3 cun along the margin of the bone or above and below the scars	Regional distending pain

Fuliu (KI-7, on the affected side)	No. 30 filiform needle, 1.5 cun in length	Insert perpendicularly to a depth of 0.5-1.0 cun	Regional distending pain or pain radiating to the sole
Fuyang (BL-59, on the affected side)	No. 30 filiform needle, 2 cun in length	Insert perpendicularly to a depth of 1.0-1.5 cun	Regional distending pain

Method
- The patient lies in a prone position.
- The acupoints are needled using electro-acupuncture, with the needles being retained for 40 minutes; during this period, one session of needle manipulation is carried out.
- After the needles are withdrawn, cupping therapy is performed for one minute.
- Acupuncture should be performed once a day; one course of treatment consists of ten sessions.
- An interval of five days is required between two courses of treatment.

Clinical notes
The effects of electro-acupuncture depend on the degree of repair achieved in the treatment of the ruptured Achilles tendon. The further advanced the repair, the better the curative effect will be. Electro-acupuncture therapy is effective in restoring the function of the calf muscle, in absorbing or softening local scars, and more especially in relieving local swelling and pain.

63 PERITENDINITIS OF THE ACHILLES TENDON

This condition is mainly caused by trauma and strain, resulting in inflammation of the Achilles tendon, the surrounding tissues and the bursa deep to the tendon.

The injury can be classified into acute and chronic forms. Sudden contusion or sprain of the Achilles tendon caused by pressure, trampolining, or running and jumping result in congestion and oedema of the tendon and surrounding tissues in the acute stage. Chronic inflammation is caused by repeated friction of the tendon and surrounding tissues, particularly from long-distance running or walking.

Both acute and chronic injury may result in degeneration of the tendon, thickening of the tendon, local adhesions or even bursitis on the calcaneus deep to the tendon.

Clinical manifestations
- in acute cases, painful swelling can be felt in the Achilles tendon immediately after injury
- appropriate treatment may relieve the pain in about a week, but inappropriate treatment may result in the condition becoming chronic
- in chronic cases, there may be no obvious swelling over the affected region
- pain gradually appears around the tendon (exacerbated by walking and jumping), with tender fusiform thickening of the tendon
- palpable crepitus around the tendon when flexing and extending the ankle

TREATMENT
Acupoints and techniques

Combination of points	Needles used	Insertion technique	Needling sensation
Tender area (on the affected side): Two obvious tender areas can be located on the medial and lateral sides over the tendo calcaneus	Two no. 30 filiform needles, 1.5 cun in length	Insert to a depth of 1.3 cun along the margin of the bone towards the opposite side of the ankle	Regional distending pain

Fuliu (KI-7, on the affected side)	No. 30 filiform needle, 1.5 cun in length	Insert perpendicularly to a depth of 0.5-1.0 cun	Regional distending pain or pain radiating to the sole
Fuyang (BL-59, on the affected side)	No. 30 filiform needle, 2 cun in length	Insert perpendicularly to a depth of 1.0-1.5 cun	Regional distending pain

Method
- The patient lies in a prone position.
- The acupoints are needled, with the needles being retained for 40 minutes; during this period, one session of needle manipulation is carried out.
- After the needles are withdrawn, cupping therapy is performed for one minute.
- Acupuncture should be performed once a day; one course of treatment consists of ten sessions.
- If the treatment is ineffective, corticosteroid injection can be considered.

Clinical notes
Acupuncture therapy is reasonably effective in treating acute peritendinitis of the Achilles tendon at an early stage. However, it is not so effective in treating chronic injury or strain, which can be dealt with satisfactorily by corticosteroid injection deep to the tendon. (Injection of corticosteroid into the Achilles tendon weakens the tendon and may result in rupture.) Regional pain may appear about 24 hours after corticosteroid injection. Patients should be warned to expect this. Acupuncture or corticosteroid injection is generally a satisfactory therapeutic method for treating this condition.

Appendix: Location of acupuncture points referred to in the book

Lung Meridian, LU 149

LU-1	Zhongfu
LU-2	Yunmen
LU-3	Tianfu
LU-7	Lieque
LU-10	Yuji

Large Intestine Meridian, LI 150

LI-4	Hegu
LI-5	Yangxi
LI-10	Shousanli
LI-11	Quchi
LI-13	Shouwuli
LI-15	Jianyu

Stomach Meridian, ST 151

ST-7	Xiaguan
ST-8	Touwei
ST-31	Biguan
ST-32	Futu
ST-35	Dubi
ST-36	Zusanli
ST-38	Tiaokou
ST-43	Xiangu

Spleen Meridian, SP 152

SP-6	Sanyinjiao
SP-9	Yinlingquan
SP-10	Xuehai
SP-12	Chongmen
SP-13	Fushe

Heart Meridian, HT 153

HT-2	Qingling
HT-3	Shaohai
HT-7	Shenmen

Small Intestine Meridian, SI 154

SI-3	Houxi
SI-5	Yanggu
SI-6	Yanglao
SI-9	Jianzhen
SI-10	Naoshu
SI-15	Jianzhongshu
SI-16	Tianchuang
SI-17	Tianrong

Bladder Meridian, BL 155

BL-23	Shenshu
BL-24	Qihaishu
BL-25	Dachangshu
BL-36	Chengfu
BL-37	Yinmen
BL-39	Weiyang
BL-40	Weizhong
BL-54	Zhibian
BL-56	Chengjin
BL-57	Chengshan
BL-59	Fuyang
BL-60	Kunlun
BL-62	Shenmai

Kidney Meridian, KI 156

KI-2	Rangu

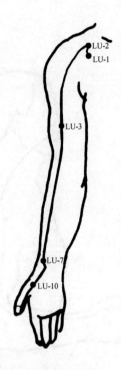

Points of Lung Meridian, LU

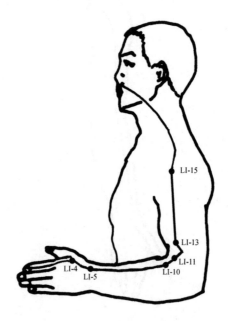

Points of Large Intestine Meridian, LI

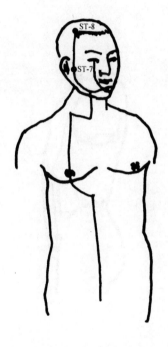
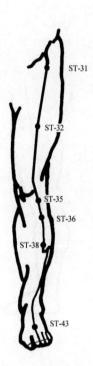

Points of Stomach Meridian, ST

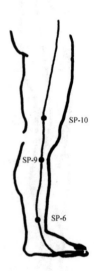

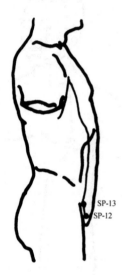

Points of Spleen Meridian, SP

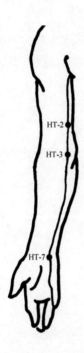

Points of Heart Meridian, HT

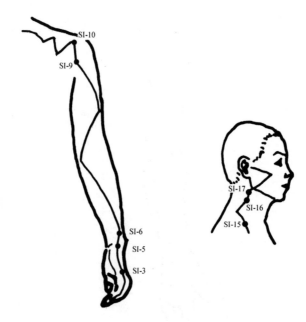

Points of Small Intestine Meridian, SI

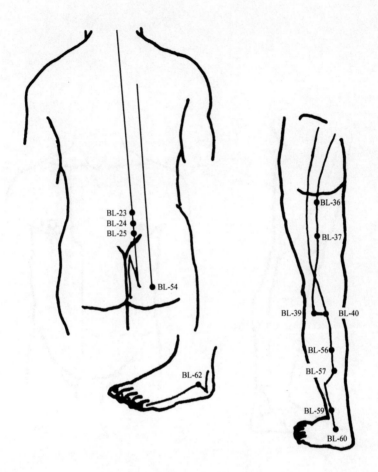

Points of Bladder Meridian, BL

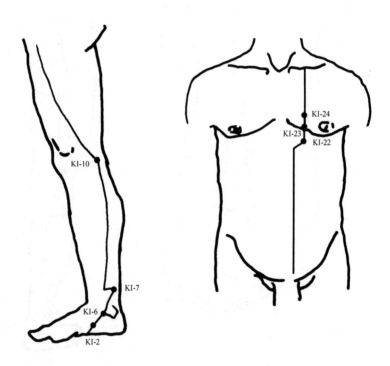

Points of Kidney Meridian, KI

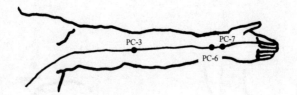

Points of Pericardium Meridian, PC

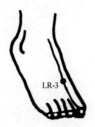

Points of Liver Meridian, LR

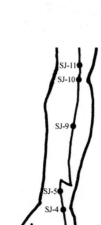
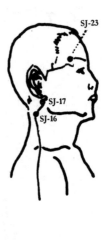

Points of Sanjiao Meridian, SJ

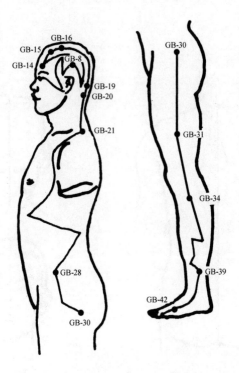

Points of Gallbladder Meridian, GB

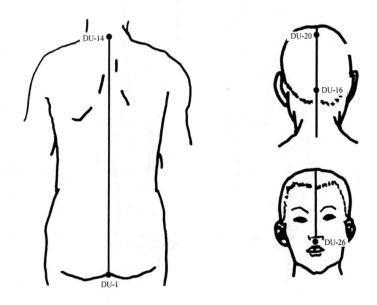

Points of Du (Governor Vessel) Meridian, DU

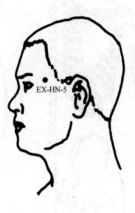

Extra Points Head and Neck, EX-HN

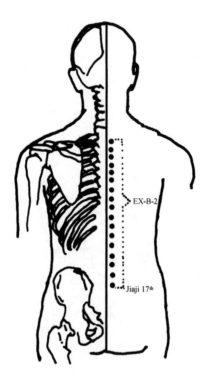

EX-B-2

Jiaji 17th

Extra Points Back, EX-B

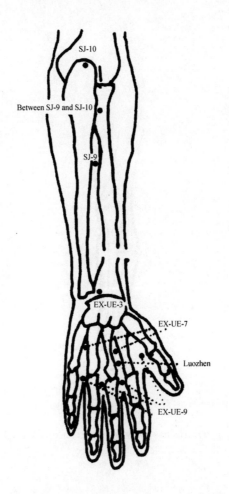

Extra Points Upper Extremities, EX-UE

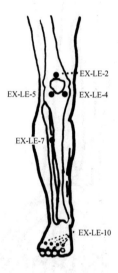

Extra Points Lower Extremities, EX-LE

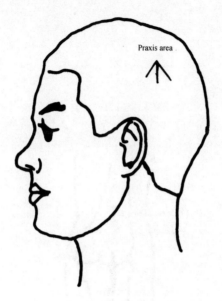

Praxis area

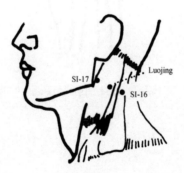

Luojing

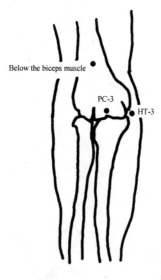

Below the biceps muscle

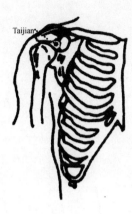

Taijian

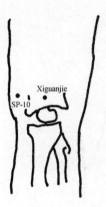

Xiguanjie

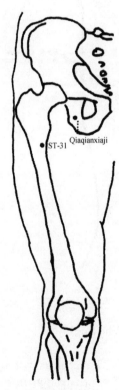

Qiaqianxiaji

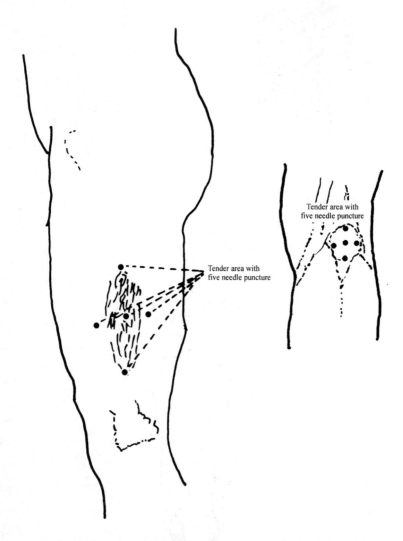

Tender area with
five needle puncture

Tender area with
five needle puncture

I Lateral aspect of the thigh   II Popliteal fossa

Tender areas with five
needle puncture

Bibliography

Chinese Academy of Traditional Chinese Medicine, *Atlas of Standard Acupuncture Points*, Qingdao: Qingdao Publishing House, 1991.

Fu Qiang, *Complete Clinical Acupuncture*, Beijing: China Medicine and Pharmaceutical Publishing House, 1991.

Hu Ximing, *Complete Secret Formulae in Traditional Chinese Medicine*, Beijing: Cultural Press, 1991.

Lu Shoukang, *Complete Practical Acupuncture*, Shanghai: Shanghai Science and Technology Publishing House, 1993.

Pan Zhiqiang, *Orthopaedic and Traumatology Handbook*, Beijing: Traditional Chinese Medicine Publishing House, 1991.

Tang Bangjie, *Orthopaedics in Traditional Chinese Medicine*, Changsha: Hunan Science and Technology Publishing House, 1988.

Wang Xuetai, *Complete Chinese Acupuncture*, Zhengzhou: Henan Science and Technology Publishing House, 1992.

Zhang Anzhen, *Orthopaedics and Traumatology in Traditional Chinese Medicine*, Beijing: People's Medical Publishing House, 1990.

Zhang Junjian, *Current Progress in Clinical Diagnosis and Treatment of Pain*, Taiyuan: Shanxi Union University Press, 1994.

Zhang Xibin, *Chinese Orthopaedics and Traumatology*, Chengdu: Sichuan Science and Technology Publishing House, 1991.

Index

the popliteal fossa, 52
the popliteal region, 58
restricted to prepatellar bursa, 120
severe in the shoulder, 66
spreading from the waist to the
popliteal fossa, 54
when bending the waist, 48, 60
when breathing, coughing and
sneezing, 30
when getting out of bed, 38, 48, 127
when going up or down stairs,
127, 132
when hyperextending the knee,
118
when raising the leg to climb stairs,
104
when sitting, 46, 60, 104
when the head is moved
backwards, 8
when the head is moved forwards, 8
when the head is moved to one
side, 8
when the head is turned slightly, 12
when the neck is bent, 12
while chewing, 14
worse when the shoulder is moved,
84
Painful arc syndrome, 70
Patellar tendon reflex reduced or
absent, 44
Pectoralis major muscle, damage to,
80
**Pectoralis major muscle,
injury to, 32-3**
**Peritendinitis of the Achilles
tendon, 144-5**
Phalangeal nerve, compression of, 140

Phonophobia, 20
Photophobia, 18, 20
Pigmented villonodular synovitis,
124
**Piriformis muscle syndrome,
106-7**
Pisiform bone, pressure on the
internal border, 90
Plantar nerves, impairment of, 138
Plantar pain, 140-1
Pleural lesion, 24
Polyuria, 20
Popliteal cyst, 122-3
Popliteal fossa, cystic swelling in,
122
Posterior tibial nerve
compression of, 138
impairment in the sensory
branches, 138
Prepatellar bursitis, 120-1
**Prolapse of the lumbar
intervertebral disc, 40-3**
Psoas major muscle, 28, 44
Ptosis, 18

Quadriceps femoris, 114
**Quadriceps femoris, sprain of,
114-15**
Quadriceps muscle
atrophy of, 44, 45
weakness of, 44

Radial nerve
injury to, 64
pressure on, 74
Radial styloid process, tender area at
the tip of, 92

Supinator, impaired function of, 74
Suppurative arthritis, 124, 126
Suppurative bursitis, 120
Supraspinatus muscle
    chronic inflammation of the
        tendon of, 70
    distending pain over, 70
Supraspinatus tendinitis, 70-1
Supraspinatus tendon, calcification
    of, 70
**Supraspinous ligament injury,
    38-9**
Synovial bursitis of the hip, 56-7

Talar tilt, 136
Tarsal tunnel syndrome, 138-9
Teichopsia, 20
**Temporomandibular joint,
    disorders of, 14-15**
Tenderness
    on greater tuberosity of the
        humerus, 70
    on the origin of the deltoid muscle,
        70
**Tendinitis of the forearm extensor
    muscles, 72-3**
Tendon of the popliteus muscle,
    damage to, 129
Tennis elbow, 78-9
**Tenovaginitis of the digital flexor
    muscles, 98-9**
Tension headache, 16-17
Tension of muscles around the
    shoulder and clavicle, 68
Thenar eminence, atrophy of, 94
**Third lumbar transverse process,
    syndrome of, 48-9**

Thoracic movement, 30
Thoracic vertebrae
    4th-6th, 38
    osteophytosis of, 24
**Thoracic vertebral joints,
    disorder of, 28-9**
Thorax
    difficulty in relaxing anterior part,
        30
    extensive bending of, 28
Thumb tendons, swelling along the
    course of, 92
Thumb
    injury to the extensor tendons of,
        72
    restriction of extension, 74
**Tibial collateral ligament of the
    knee, injury to, 127-8**
Tietze's syndrome, 34-5
Tinnitus, 14
Trapezius muscle, 8, 10, 28, 70
**Traumatic synovitis of the
    knee, 124-6**
**Triangular cartilage,
    injury to, 96-7**
Triceps muscle, rupture of the
    tendon of, 76
Triceps surae muscle, weakness and
    atrophy of, 142
Trochanteric bursitis, 108-9
Tuberculous arthritis, 124
Tumour, 24

**Ulnar nerve compression,
    90-1**
Ulnar nerve, pressure on, 90
Upper arm, overstrain of, 32